THE COMPLETE KETOGENIC DIET TO LOSE WEIGHT:

A 30-Day Meal Plan and Tasty, Easy Recipes to Experience All the Benefits of The Ketogenic Diet. A Comprehensive Guide That Even Dummies Can Follow.

© Copyright 2020 - all rights reserved.

Table Of Contents

Introduction

The keto diet is getting more and more popular these days. Is it something you would be considering for yourself? Are you just looking for a natural way to reach your goal weight? If you are, then maybe the keto diet is for you! The keto diet first became popular as a treatment for epilepsy and diabetes. People were finding that replacing their carb intake with fats helped their brain chemistry reach a steadier state. Many people found that the keto diet helped their energy levels, helped them lose weight, and helped improve their mental function.

The keto diet is completely different than most diets out there. This is a diet that is based on carbohydrates, protein and fats. Most diets are based around these three things but with the keto diet, fat is going to be your focus. The keto diet dictates that you have to consume fat 90% of the time. Fat can be in the form of oils, nuts, natural butter, or even avocados. You will be eating very limited amounts of protein and carbohydrates. Don't be alarmed! It's not too bad, we promise!

Keto recipes have become one of the most popular things in any healthy living circles. There are a lot of people who are on keto diet and continue to research on more and more keto recipes and come up with new keto recipes every day in order to keep their diet interesting.

Keto diet became famous from trend diets in the last few years. This book is a compilation of different recipes for Keto diet.

Unlike other diet books, this book also provides you with a ketogenic meal plan. This means that you could follow the recipes to the T and get the results that you want.

Short on time? With other diet books, you might be wondering when you should have some carbs on the top of your breakfast and lunch. This book has a meal plan which has you have some carbs in the morning and certain carbs in the afternoon.

What is the recipe for?

This book's purpose is to provide you with a wide variety of recipes that you can use leading up to the start of the keto diet. This book also provides you with a full day meal plan.

When you are getting started with keto, it's nice to have some variety. The best part is, these keto recipes are all healthy! The main thing to remember is that you're cutting out carbs in order to get the full benefits of the keto diet. You can't just be eating sandwiches and wings all the time.

What will you be fiddling?

This book contains a collection of high-quality recipes from a wide variety of cuisines.

No matter which one you choose, it's bound to be healthy and something you will enjoy eating.

Taking the time to browse through this book will give you a wide variety of options to choose from. Make sure you bookmark this page for later.

Carbs in Keto – The Benefits

Carbs are one of the basic necessities of our body. Carbs keep us going! Without them, we wouldn't be able to do anything! As much as we love to have carbs, however, they come with a lot of ill effects. If you take a look at something called a Ketogenic diet, you will notice that most of them is based on fat, not carbs. A lot of people have found themselves having better health, weight loss, and increased energy from following a diet that is low in carbs. Instead of replacing the carbs with fat, many people opted to replace the carbs with proteins. This made it easier to stay in ketosis.

Many studies in the medical field have shown that carbohydrate intake does not mean that weight gain is caused. This is because those carbs have to be burned off before they can result in weight gain. If the carbs are not being burned off, the body will store them as fat for future use!

There is also another reason for cutting carbs on a Keto diet. If you are following the diet, you will get used to burning fat for energy. Keeping in mind that most of the carbs are being burnt off, you will be burning fat for an extended period of time. So, your process of going into ketosis will be extended. This proves to be more effective, not only when you are trying to lose weight.

What are the Benefits of the keto diet?

- Helps in-spite weight
- Helps in-spite weight Helps in improving your body image
- Helps in improving your body image Reduces inflammation

- Reduces inflammation Increases protein turnover
- Increases protein turnover Helps in healthy metabolism
- Helps in healthy metabolism Improves insulin sensitivity
- Improves insulin sensitivity Improves physical and mental performance
- Improves physical and mental performance Improves cardiovascular health
- Improves cardiovascular health Improves athletic performance

As you can see, the Ketogenic diet has some pretty amazing benefits. You can also see that they can help you lead a happier, healthier and more active lifestyle. The benefits are not only mental and physical, but they are short-term and long-term too. It's almost like a win-win situation.

The Keto Diet – Let's Get Started

The first step is to decide whether or not you are going to try the Keto diet. You might know the benefits that come with a Keto diet, but you might also want to consider the cons. When you are considering the cons, you need to consider whether or not you are willing to make some decent adjustments to your lifestyle. If you do get going and make those changes, in the long run, it will be worth it.

Imagine yourself in the future, years after you start the diet. Everything has become normal for you. You can eat foods like pizza, cheese, bacon, drinking soda, and even eating whole wheat bread. You don't even need to think about what you are going to eat for dinner.

On the other hand, you might not want to give up your favorite foods and hide everything you eat. However, if you do decide to follow a keto diet, it would be best if you start with those that are unhealthy.

CHAPTER 1:

The Ketogenic Diet and Lifestyle to Follow

Keto or ketogenic diet is simply a "low carb diet," with a high fat and protein consumption. The Keto diet is often considered to be the same as the Atkin diet. However, they are different. The difference between the two is in the amount of protein consumed.

Another difference is that the keto diet puts the body in ketosis throughout the whole stage. Nevertheless, the Atkin diet only puts the body in ketosis during the first and probably the second phase.

At times, we recommend the ketogenic diet for treating specific ailments. For example, the keto diet can help control diabetes. Also, since the 19th century, the keto diet has been used to treat epilepsy in children.

One of the gaining uses of the keto diet is for weight loss. However, there are other low carb diets that you can use for weight loss. Common examples of such diets are South Beach, Dukan, and Paleo diets. What makes the keto diet stands out is fat composition, which is usually between 55-60%.

The word keto is derived from ketosis, which is a natural metabolic process. We can say that a Ketogenic diet is that combination of meal which can induce or accelerate the rate of ketosis occurring in the human body. The next argument would be why ketosis is considered healthy? Ketosis is the process in which fats are broken down to release energy and ketones. It benefits by producing a fair amount of energy, reducing the body's stored fats, and providing ketones for body metabolism. It is noteworthy that ketosis cannot occur in freely available glucose or Carbohydrates: in the body. Our usual diet contains more carbohydrates than fats; we naturally rely on carbohydrates to extract the required energy. The ketogenic diet is the way of shifting our carb driven body to a fat driven one. Doing so restricts the daily carb intake to 50grams and recommends a fair use of fats instead. All high carbohydrates ingredients are forbidden in this diet plan.

Less sugar intake means lowering the toxic agents in the blood. The same toxins are responsible for causing acne and other skin problems. The ketogenic diet is, therefore, proving to be effective in controlling acne.

When a ketogenic diet was studied to find any prevention or cure for certain types of cancer, the studies suggested that it can indeed be used as a complementary treatment for people who are on chemo and radiotherapy. The ketogenic diet can increase the cancerous cells' oxidative stress more than the normal cells, and hence they can be easily destroyed.

When the ketogenic dieters make health choices and consume high and good fats, contain high-density lipoprotein- HDL. These cholesterols can attach to the bad cholesterol and then removed from the body.

When the cholesterol is no longer deposited in the blood vessel, the heart condition will gradually improve.

This high-fat diet is most effective in boosting brain functioning. As the fats are nourishing for the brain cells and the diet also detoxifies the neurons. This factor is why a ketogenic diet is highly recommended to people with Alzheimer's, Epilepsy, and memory loss.

One added advantage of a ketogenic diet is that people with epilepsy can control their seizures. PCOS or Polycystic ovarian syndrome is a medical condition that can bring adverse health effects to a woman. And it is a known fact that a high carb diet further aggravates this condition's damaging effects. Therefore, a ketogenic diet can be used to counter those effects.

The ketogenic diet reduces your carbohydrate consumption while promoting high fat intake—protein consumption in moderation. The extreme restriction it puts on carbohydrate consumption may make the ketogenic diet seem like a carb-restrictive diet, but that's not the case. The actual goal of this diet is to encourage a state called "ketosis." Ketosis occurs when the body starts using fats as a primary source of fuel instead of using glucose. Fats are then metabolized for producing ketones. Ketosis happens when your body doesn't have enough glucose.

Glucose is known to create an instant high in the body, followed by a sudden crash. It results in a high level of functioning in the brain, followed by a sudden decline. That's why people who consume high-fat diets experience frequent brain fogs, which hinder their capacity to concentrate on a particular subject.

On the other hand, the ketone bodies offer a constant supply of energy without causing any disruption. It is especially beneficial for tissues like the heart and the brain.

The keto diet has become so popular in recent years because of the success people have noticed. Not only have they managed to lose weight, but scientific studies show that the keto diet can help you improve your health in many others. As when starting any new diet or exercise routine, there may seem to be some disadvantages, so we will go over those for the keto diet. But most people agree that the benefits outweigh the adjustment period!

Helps You Lose Weight

For most people, this is the first and foremost benefit of switching to keto! Their former diet method may have stalled for them, or they were starting to notice weight creeping back on. With keto, studies have shown that people have been able to follow this diet and relay fewer hunger pangs and suppressed appetite while losing weight at the same time! You are minimizing your carbohydrate intake, which means less blood sugar spikes. Those fluctuations in blood sugar levels often make you feel hungrier and prone to snacking in between meals. Instead, by guiding the body towards ketosis, you eat a more fulfilling diet of fat and protein and harnessing energy from ketone molecules instead of glucose. Studies show that low carb diets effectively reduce visceral fat (the type of fat you commonly see around the abdomen that increases as you become overweight and obese). It reduces your risk of obesity and improves your health in the long run.

Decreases Risk of Type 2 Diabetes

The problem with carbohydrates is how unstable they make blood sugar levels. It can be hazardous for people who have diabetes or are considered pre-diabetic due to varying blood sugar levels or family history. Keto is an excellent option because of the minimal intake of carbohydrates it requires. Instead, you are harnessing most of your calories from fat or protein, which will not cause blood sugar spikes and ultimately put less pressure on the pancreas to secrete insulin. Many studies have found that diabetes patients who followed the keto diet lost more weight and eventually reduced their fasting glucose levels. It is excellent news for patients who have unstable blood sugar levels or hope to avoid or reduce their diabetes medication intake.

Lower Your Chances of Having Heart Disease

Most people assume that following a keto that is so high in fat content increases your risk of coronary heart disease or heart attack. But the research proves otherwise! Research shows that switching to keto can lower your blood pressure, increase your HDL good cholesterol, and reduce your triglyceride fatty acid levels. That's because the fats you consume on keto are healthy and high-quality fats, which tends to reverse many unhealthy symptoms of heart disease and boost your "good" HDL cholesterol numbers and decrease your "bad" LDL cholesterol numbers. It also reduces the level of triglyceride fatty acids in the bloodstream. A high level of these can lead to stroke, heart attack, or premature death. And what are the high levels of fatty acids linked? Increased consumption of carbohydrates.

With the keto diet, you are drastically cutting your carbohydrates intake to improve fatty acid levels and improve other risk factors. A 2018 study on the keto diet found that it can improve as many as 22 out of 26 risk factors for cardiovascular heart disease! These factors can be crucial to some people, especially those with a history of heart disease in their family.

Increase Our Body Energy Levels

We compared the glucose molecules' difference synthesized from a high carbohydrate intake versus ketones produced on the keto diet. Ketones are produced by the liver and use fat molecules you already have stored. It makes them much more energy-rich and an endless fuel source than glucose, a simple sugar molecule.

These ketones can physically and mentally give you a burst of energy, allowing you to have greater focus, clarity, and attention to detail.

Decreases Inflammation in The Body

Inflammation on its own is a natural response by the body's immune system, but when it becomes uncontrollable, it can lead to an array of health problems, some severe, some minor.

The many health concerns include acne, autoimmune conditions, arthritis, psoriasis, irritable bowel syndrome, and even acne and eczema. Often, removing sugars and carbohydrates from your diet can help patients of these diseases avoid flare-ups - and the good news is keto does just that!

A 2008 research study found that keto decreased a blood marker linked to high body inflammation by nearly 40%. It is excellent news for people who may suffer from inflammatory disease and is willing to change their diet to see improvement hopefully.

Increases Your Mental Functioning Level

Like we elaborated earlier, energy-rich ketones can boost the body's physical and mental levels of alertness.

Research has shown that keto is a much better energy source for the brain than simple sugar glucose molecules are. With nearly 75% of your diet coming from healthy fats, the brain's neural cells and mitochondria have a better energy source to function at the highest level. Some studies have tested patients on the keto diet and found they had higher cognitive functioning, better memory recall, and less memory loss. The keto diet can even decrease the occurrence of migraines, which can be very detrimental to patients.

Decreases Risk of Diseases Like Alzheimer's, Parkinson's, And Epilepsy.

The keto diet was created in the 1920s as a way to combat Epilepsy in children. From there, research has found that keto can improve your cognitive functioning level and protect brain cells from injury or damage. This discovery reduces neurodegenerative disease risk, which begins in the brain due to neural cells mutating and functioning with damaged parts or lower than peak optimal functioning.

Studies have found that the following keto can improve patients' mental functioning who suffer from Alzheimer's or Parkinson's.

These neurodegenerative diseases sadly have no cure, but the keto diet could improve symptoms as they progress. Researchers believe that is due to cutting out carbs from your diet, which reduces blood sugar spikes that the body's neural cells have to adjust continually.

Can Regulate Hormones in Women Who Have PCOS and PMS

Women who have PCOS (polycystic ovary syndrome) have infertility, which can be heartbreaking for young couples trying to start a family. There is no cure for this condition, but it is believed to be related to many similar diabetic symptoms like obesity and high insulin levels. It causes the body to produce more sex hormones, which can lead to infertility. The keto diet has become a popular method to regulate insulin and hormone levels and increase women's chances of getting pregnant.

CHAPTER 2:

Food Recommendations and Food to Avoid

Food can get complicated. There are so many different classifications filled with various types filled with subsets; it's a lot to process. Understanding food can be the basic building block to starting a specific diet, though. If a person doesn't understand how a particular food affects their body, they might be less inclined to follow the diet or confused about why one cheat day can throw off their whole body. The kind of foods and the nourishments we obtained from it directly impacts the body's functions. Just like people can enjoy having a routine, the body also has a routine throughout the day, knowing what kind of food to expect.

Keto can take a body's natural routine and throw it into a tailspin for a few days. Though, pushing through this period can show just how much the food people choose to eat can affect their bodies. Certain foods are broken down can determine if they will cause someone to gain or lose weight. There is a long list of traditionally thought foods to help people lose weight that is also keto-approved.

Weighted Portions

It is no mystery that the food people eat can contribute to weight fluctuations. It is usually the first thing people adjust and exercise when they want to lose weight. It is not by accident.

The types of food people consume directly impact their physical health and how their body works internally.

Most people look to portion control and increasing exercise as the perfect recipe for weight loss. It can yield results over time but can also be frustrating and time-consuming. When people start these regiments, they sometimes don't use a guide and decide to eat better food without determining their goals. Cutting out the right kinds of foods is the key to weight loss. The biggest culprit for weight gain is carbohydrates. People often attempt to cut down the number of carbs they eat but don't think about the type of carbs. For example, a piece of bread is a dense slab of carbs that is hard for the body to break down, but a stalk of broccoli is low in carbs and easy for the stomach to break down for energy.

Things like bread and crackers are also often filled with added sugars. It means that the body will have to break down the sugar derived from carbohydrates and the added extra sugar. It takes a lot of time and energy and, when there is excess sugar, it is stored away in the body as fat.

Diets that are high in carbs and low in fats and fiber can cause other difficulties as well. Without enough fat or fiber, there is nothing in the body to absorb the glucose being produced, so most of it is sent into the bloodstream. It can cause spikes and crashes in people's blood sugar levels. Besides, when blood sugar spikes, it triggers increased insulin production in the pancreas. This hormone turns sugar into fat, but too much in someone's system can cause diabetes.

With grains making up the most Western diet, it can be challenging for people to pull away from carbs. Looking at a traditionally considered food list to help people lose weight can help them change their perspective. It is not a coincidence either that most foods that make up these lists are also keto-approved.

The first food on this list is one of the main keto staples: eggs. Eggs are high in protein and fat, making them a filling meal all on their own. They can also help with balancing cholesterol levels and are easy to be creative with because there are so many ways to cook them.

Next in line are dark leafy greens, low in carbs and packed with fiber, vitamin K, and other minerals people need. These are great to pick up in the grocery store for salads or lettuce wraps or cook down in oil for a salty afternoon snack or soup. Other approved vegetables are in the cruciferous family. These include broccoli, cauliflower, cabbage, and Brussels sprouts. They all are packed with fiber and a little bit of protein to make satisfying snacks that are simple for the body to break down and use as energy.

Moving over to proteins, one of the standard healthy options is salmon. Salmon is full of omega-3 fatty acids, which bodies love, and it also contains a considerable amount of protein. These benefits are not restricted to salmon, though. People can find these qualities in most fatty fish, such as tuna, shrimp, crab, cod, and more. At the meat counter, proteins that are considered traditionally healthy are lean meats and chicken.

Chicken is an excellent source of clean protein that can help burn calories as it's digested. Although people on regular diets might focus on eating lean cuts of red meat, people on keto should look for the fattier cuts to fuel their bodies.

Carbohydrates and Fat Content

When eating foods on a keto-based diet, people consume mostly fats to train their liver to use that source as energy instead of glucose. It is a process the liver is not used to and is not its default; it only reverts to this emergency process. However, by adjusting their diet contents, a person can completely change how their liver functions.

Typically, the liver helps to break down food into sugars and then turns extra sugar into fat for storing. It is how it likes to do its job. However, on the keto diet, people use the food they eat to coax their liver into operating a different way. When deprived of things that it can turn into sugar, the liver is forced to use fat as energy. It will pull from the storage pockets of fat first, then use the fat it is fed to turn into ketones that the body will use for energy.

This process also affects insulin production because that is the hormone used to turn sugar into fat. If there is no sugar in the body, the pancreas will not produce as much insulin because it is not needed. It can benefit people with diabetes or high blood sugar to regulate their symptoms.

Once the liver starts creating ketones and all of the glucose has been purged, a person's body will begin using the ketones as energy on its own. Ketones are especially interesting because, like glucose, they can cross the blood-brain barrier and act as fuel for the brain and the body. Even when the body is running on ketones, that doesn't mean its preferences have changed. People need to remember that their body will always prefer to run on sugar, so having a cheat day loaded with carbs can potentially pull them out of ketosis. Constant diligence is required to keep a keto body because it all depends on the food a person eats.

It might be surprising to some that fats can have such a drastic impact on the body. They are a large group with many different types and characteristics, so their effect on the body can be broad. Their presence is undoubtedly essential, though. The body uses fats as a kind of storage facility for energy. In situations where it is low on glucose or carbs, it can pull from pockets of fat and process that for energy in a pinch. Fat also helps to insulate the body, so it stays warm in cold weather, and it protects the organs from any potential damage during day-to-day life.

Fats also help the body break down proteins and harvest energy from their parts. They start chemical reactions throughout the body that can help people grow, improve immune system health and function, and start the metabolic process of breaking down all foods. Fats are also great at storing nutrients. They frequently help to store a range of vitamins in the body, including vitamins A, D, E, and K. These vitamins are referred to as fat-soluble vitamins for this reason. Having reserves of key nutrients like these is like an insurance policy for the body that it will never be completely depleted of anything it needs to operate.

The three most common types of fats are LDL (low-density lipoproteins), HDL (high-density lipoproteins), and triglycerides.

Several other types of fats fit under the category of lipids. LDL and HDL fats are what is measured when finding someone's cholesterol levels.

Triglycerides are the primary type of fat that people consume through food because the body does not produce high levels of this on its own. These fats can provide more than twice as much energy as carbs or proteins can on their own, making it a powerhouse for keto dieters. Choosing to eat more of these fatty foods can be beneficial not only because they provide more energy to the body but also because eating more fats can mean decreasing sugar intake. It is causing a long list of health issues on its own.

CHAPTER 3:

Tips for Losing Weight Quickly with Ketogenic Diet

The ketogenic diet refers to a high-fat, moderate protein, and low-carb meal plan. The diet is also referred to as a low-carb diet or low-carb high-fat diet. In this diet, you get 70 to 75% of your calories from fat. You also obtain 20 to 25% from proteins and the remaining 5 to 10% from carbohydrates. Once you start following this way of eating, many health benefits start accruing to your body ranging from weight loss to proper management of type 2 diabetics. Alongside this, you also get to enjoy a steady supply of energy, more focus, and mental clarity, etc.

A Carbohydrate-Rich Diet

To comprehend more about the ketogenic diet and its principles, you need to get a picture of what happens in the human body when you take food on a carbohydrate-rich diet.

When the food is broken down, glucose and insulin are released by the body. Since glucose is the most accessible energy source for the body to use, it prefers other sources. What's more, insulin is produced to transport glucose to different parts of the body through the bloodstream. Meanwhile, fat gets stored.

Next, let us see what happens when carbohydrate consumption is drastically cut in the ketogenic diet. When there is a severe reduction of carb intake accompanied by increased fat consumption, the body undergoes a metabolic state known as ketosis. Ketosis is the end goal of a properly maintained ketogenic diet. Once the body is in ketosis, fat molecules get burned for energy instead of carbohydrates. In simple words, it means that your body will be burning fat for fuel or energy instead of carbohydrates. During ketosis, ketones are released from the liver to the bloodstreams.

Ketones are an alternative fuel energy source that the liver produces from the fat stored in the body. As a result of all these, insulin levels get severely reduced in the blood. And fat gets to be used effectively.

Since you clearly understand the basics, let us move advance forward and know what you can consume in the ketogenic diet and what needs to be avoided. We will try to understand the benefits that are offered when you are following the ketogenic diet.

Ease into the Ketogenic Diet Slowly and Gradually

Rather than going head straight into the diet by avoiding all carbs rich foods, choose a few carb-rich foods you can forego more easily. Transitioning at one go can be hard and impossible to get through, especially during the initial days.

So, try avoiding a few carbs rich foods items at each phase and slowly get into the eating plan.

Proper Planning & Meal Plan

Planning plays a significant role in the success of the ketogenic diet. Without proper planning, it becomes easier to fall through for the temptations. Have a diet plan ready at all times.

Reduced Consumption of Carbohydrates

Make sure to restrict the amount of carbohydrate intake per day to less than 20gm once you have got settled into the diet plan. The lower the level of carbs, the faster you get into ketosis. Net carbs should be less than 20gm, and total carbs should be less than 30gm per day.

Increased Consumption of Fat

Increase the intake of fat-rich food and a moderate amount of protein so that you can feel satiated and fuller for a longer duration of time. Avoid binging on foods as it can slow ketosis and thereby the progression into the diet.

Moderate Consumption of Proteins

Do not over consume proteins. An ideal protein consumption ratio is about 1.2 to 1.7gm of proteins per kilogram of reference body weight per day.

Higher Intake of Water

Make sure to drink a suitable amount of water to keep dehydration at bay since ketosis can sometimes make you feel thirsty. Aim for anything between 1o to 16 cups of water.

Regular Physical Exercise

Undertaking exercise can lower the level of carbohydrates while increasing the levels of ketones. Exercising for about 15 to 30 minutes would be fine.

Intake of Electrolytes

Taking a broth or bouillon cup during the initial days is an excellent idea to reduce keto flu symptoms. Or you can salt your food liberally. Taking an acceptable amount of water and electrolytes together is essential.

Clearing Off & Refurbishing the Pantry

Before you start the diet, make sure to remove all the food items which are rich in carbohydrates from your pantry. And fill it with keto essential pantry items.

A Proper Check of Labels

Always check labels and ingredients list of all food items to ensure no hidden ingredients rich in sugar or carbohydrates—for example, dextrose, etc.

CHAPTER 4:

30-Day Program

Day	Breakfast	Snack	Lunch	Snack	Dinner
1	Peanut Butter Cup Smoothie	Butter Slow-Cooker Mushrooms	Lime Chicken with Savoy Cabbage	Moist Avocado Brownies	Grilled Leg of Lamb
2	Berry Green Smoothie	Baked Zucchini Gratin	Middle Eastern Lamb Zucchini Casserole	Choco Peanut Cookies	Herb-Simmered Beef Stew
3	Lemon-Cashew Smoothie	Roasted Radishes with Brown Butter Sauce	Ginger Steak Broccoli	Maple and Pecan Bars	Sesame and Chorizo Cauliflower Rice

4	Spinach-Blueberry Smoothie	Parmesan and Pork Rind Green Beans	BLT Chicken Salad	Chocolate Cupcakes	Cheddar Zucchini & Beef Mugs
5	Nut Medley Granola	Pesto Cauliflower Steaks	Figs and Goat Cheese-Stuffed Chicken	Chocolate Chip Mug Cake	Grilled Beef Short Loin
6	Bacon-Artichoke Omelet	Tomato, Avocado, and Cucumber Salad	Carne Asada	Creamy Coconut Hazelnut Cake	Herby Beef & Veggie Stew
7	Mushroom Frittata	Crunchy Pork Rind Zucchini Sticks	Amazing Pulled Pork	Ice Cream Brownies	Sausage with Zucchini Lasagna
8	Breakfast Bake	Cauliflower "Potato" Salad	Braised Pork Belly	Mint Brownies with Hazelnuts	Tarragon Beef Meatloaf

9	Avocado and Eggs	Loaded Cauliflower Mashed "Potatoes"	Peppercorn Short Ribs	Mocha Pots de Crème	Sausage with Tomatoes and Cheese
10	Creamy Cinnamon Smoothie	Pork Rind Nachos	Spicy Italian Sausage and Zucchini Noodles	Chocolate Chip Pudding	Sweet & Sour Pork Chops
11	Morning Buzz Iced Coffee	Sour Cream and Onion Pork Rinds	Meaty Cauliflower Lasagna	Vanilla Cherry Panna Cotta	Tuscan Pork Tenderloin with Cauli Rice
12	Frittata	Baked Cheddar Chips	Chili Verde	Orange Lime Pudding	Baked tenderloin with Lime Chimichurri
13	Green Goddess Smoothie	Baked Parmesan Chips	Pork & Bacon Parcels	Guacamole Deviled Eggs	Shitake Butter Steak

14	Blueberry Power Smoothie	Mini Mozzarella Crust Pizza	Yummy Spareribs in Bearnaise Sauce	Curry Spiced Almonds	Garlic and Lime Marinated Pork Chops
15	Spiced Oranged-Pistachio Smoothie	Mini Salami and Cheese Pizzas	Salisbury Steak	Chia Peanut Butter Bites	Zoodles with Bolognese Sauce
16	Florentine Breakfast Sandwich	Chicken Ramen Dip	Delicious Pork Stew	Cheesy Sausage Dip	Chili Zucchini Beef Lasagna
17	Avocado Toast	Creamy Crab Dip	Asian Ground Pork Bowl with Fried Eggs	Salted Kale Chips	Rib Roast with Roasted Red Shallots and Garlic
18	Baklava Hot Porridge	Bacon-Whiskey Caramelized Onion Dip	Sausage and Cheese Wrap	Bacon Jalapeno Quick Bread	Beef Ragu with a Twist

19	Greek Yogurt Parfait	Creamy Dill Deviled Eggs	Broccoli & Ground Beef Casserole	Toasted Pumpkin Seeds	Ground Pork & Scrambled Eggs with Cabbage
20	Egg Baked in Avocado	Roasted Pesto Pepper Poppers	Curry Beef	Bacon-Wrapped Burger Bites	Traditional Beef Bourguignon
21	Cheese Crepes	Macadamia Shortbread Cookies	Sprouts Stir-fry with Kale, Broccoli, and Beef	Almond Sesame Crackers	Basil Prosciutto Pizza
22	Ricotta Pancakes	Chocolate Muffins	Korean Braised Beef with Kelp Noodles	Cauliflower Cheese Dip	Keto Crispy Rosemary Chicken Drumsticks
23	Yogurt Waffles	No-Bake Coconut Cookies	Assorted Grilled Veggies & Beef Steaks	Deviled Eggs with Bacon	Baked Pesto Chicken

24	Broccoli Muffins	Coconut Blondies	Lemony Sea Bass Fillet	Coleslaw with Avocado Dressing	Low-Carb Pork Medallions
25	Pumpkin Bread	Chocolate and Hazelnut Spread	Curried Fish with Super Greens	Baked Cauliflower Bites	Bacon-Wrapped Pork Chops
26	Eggs in Avocado Cups	Cinnamon and Cardamom Fat Bombs	Shrimp Alfredo	Bacon-Wrapped Shrimp	Rosemary Chicken with Avocado Sauce
27	Cheddar Scramble	Coconut Panna Cotta with Cream & Caramel	Garlic-Lemon Mahi Mahi	Raspberry Cheesecake Fluff	Crispy Chicken Nuggets
28	Bacon Omelet	Blueberry Ice Balls	Scallops in Creamy Garlic Sauce	Keto Hot Fudge	Zucchini & Bell Pepper Chicken Gratin

29	Green Veggies Quiche	Raspberry Coconut Cheesecake	Shrimp Curry	Hot Caramel Sauce	Herb Pork Chops with Cranberry Sauce
30	Chicken & Asparagus Frittata	Avocado & Berry Fruit Dessert	Israeli Salmon Salad	5-Minute Chocolate Mousse	Pork Chops with Basil Tomato Sauce

CHAPTER 5:

Breakfast

Peanut Butter Cup Smoothie

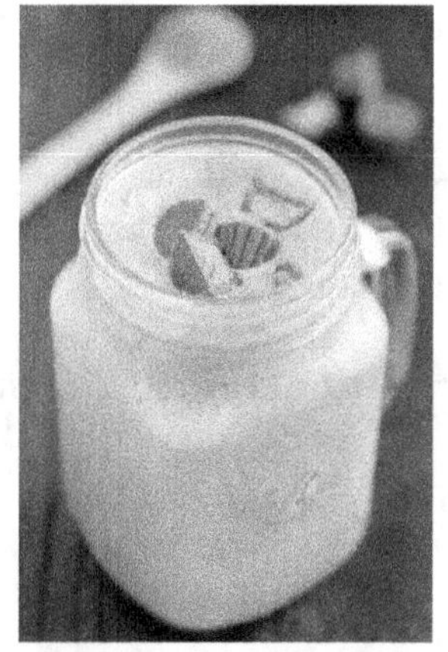

Preparation Time: 5 Minutes

Cooking Time: 0 Minutes

Servings: 2

Ingredients:

- 1 cup of water
- ¾ cup coconut cream
- One scoop chocolate protein powder
- Two tablespoons natural peanut butter
- Three ice cubes

Directions:

1. Put the water, coconut cream, protein powder, peanut butter, and ice in a blender and blend until smooth.
2. Pour into two glasses and serve immediately.

Nutrition:

Calories: 486

Fat: 40g

Protein: 30g

Carbs: 11g

Fiber: 5g

Berry Green Smoothie

Preparation Time: 10 Minutes

Cooking Time: 0 Minutes

Servings: 2

Ingredients:

- 1 cup of water
- ½ cup raspberries
- ½ cup shredded kale
- ¾ cup cream cheese
- One tablespoon coconut oil
- One scoop vanilla protein powder

Directions:

1. Put the water, raspberries, kale, cream cheese, coconut oil, and protein powder in a blender and blend until smooth.
2. Pour into two glasses and serve immediately.

Nutrition:

Calories: 436

Fat: 36g

Protein: 28g

Carbs: 11g

Fiber: 5g

Lemon-Cashew Smoothie

Preparation Time: 5 Minutes

Cooking Time: 0 Minutes

Servings: 1

Ingredients:

- 1 cup unsweetened cashew milk
- ¼ cup heavy (whipping) cream
- ¼ cup freshly squeezed lemon juice
- One scoop plain protein powder

- One tablespoon coconut oil
- One teaspoon sweetener

Directions:

1. Put the cashew milk, heavy cream, lemon juice, protein powder, coconut oil, and sweetener in a blender and blend until smooth.
2. Pour into a glass and serve immediately.

Nutrition:

Calories: 503

Fat: 45g

Protein: 29g

Carbs: 15g

Fiber: 4g

Spinach-Blueberry Smoothie

Preparation Time: 5 Minutes

Cooking Time: 0 Minutes

Servings: 2

Ingredients:

- 1 cup of coconut milk
- 1 cup spinach
- ½ English cucumber, chopped
- ½ cup blueberries
- One scoop plain protein powder
- Two tablespoons coconut oil
- Four ice cubes
- Mint sprigs, for garnish

Directions:

1. Put the coconut milk, spinach, cucumber, blueberries, protein powder, coconut oil,

and ice in a blender and blend until smooth.

2. Pour into two glasses, garnish each with the mint, and serve immediately.

Nutrition:

Calories: 353

Fat: 32g

Protein: 15g

Carbs: 9g

Fiber: 3g

Creamy Cinnamon Smoothie

Preparation Time: 5 Minutes

Cooking Time: 0 Minutes

Servings: 2

Ingredients:

- 2 cups of coconut milk
- One scoop vanilla protein powder
- 5 drops liquid stevia
- One teaspoon ground cinnamon
- ½ teaspoon alcohol-free vanilla extract

Directions:

1. Put the coconut milk, protein powder, stevia, cinnamon, and vanilla in a blender and blend until smooth.
2. Pour into two glasses and serve immediately.

Nutrition:

Calories: 492

Fat: 47g

Protein: 18g

Carbs: 8g

Fiber: 2g

Nut Medley Granola

Preparation Time: 10 Minutes

Cooking Time: 60 Minutes

Servings: 8

Ingredients:

- 2 cups shredded unsweetened coconut
- 1 cup sliced almonds
- 1 cup raw sunflower seeds
- ½ cup raw pumpkin seeds
- ½ cup walnuts
- ½ cup melted coconut oil
- 10 drops liquid stevia
- One teaspoon ground cinnamon
- ½ teaspoon ground nutmeg

Directions:

1. Preheat the oven to 250 F.
2. Line 2 baking sheets with parchment paper. Set aside.
3. Toss the shredded coconut, almonds, sunflower seeds, pumpkin seeds, and walnuts in a large bowl until mixed.
4. In a small bowl, mix the stevia, coconut oil, cinnamon, and nutmeg until mixed.
5. Pour the coconut oil combination into the nut mixture and use your hands to blend until the nuts are very well coated.
6. Put the granola mixture on the baking sheets and spread it out evenly.
7. Bake the granola, stir every 10 to 15 minutes, wait for the mixture is

golden brown and crunchy, about 1 hour.

8. Handover the granola to a large bowl and let the granola cool, tossing it frequently to break up the large pieces.

9. Store the granola in sealed containers in the refrigerator or freezer for up to 1 month.

Nutrition:

Calories: 391 Fat: 38g

Protein: 10g

Carbs: 10g

Fiber: 6g

Bacon-Artichoke Omelet

Preparation Time: 10 Minutes

Cooking Time: 10 Minutes

Servings: 4

Ingredients:

- Six eggs, beaten
- Two tablespoons heavy (whipping) cream
- Eight bacon slices, cooked and chopped
- One tablespoon olive oil
- ¼ cup chopped onion
- ½ cup chopped artichoke hearts (canned, packed in water)
- Sea salt
- Freshly ground black pepper

Directions:

1. In a small bowl, blend the eggs, heavy cream, and bacon until well blended, and set aside.

2. Place a large skillet over medium-high heat and add the olive oil.

3. Sauté the onion until tender, about 3 minutes.

4. Pour the egg mixture into the skillet, swirling it for 1 minute.

5. Cook the omelet, lifting the edges with a spatula to let the uncooked egg flow underneath, for 2 minutes.

6. Sprinkle the artichoke hearts on top and flip the omelet. Cook for 4 minutes more until the egg is firm. Flip the omelet over again, so the artichoke hearts are on top.

7. Remove from the heat, cut the omelet into quarters, and season with salt and black pepper. Transfer the omelet to plates and serve.

Nutrition:

Calories: 435

Fat: 39g

Protein: 17g

Carbs: 5g

Fiber: 2g

Mushroom Frittata

Preparation Time: 10 Minutes

Cooking Time: 15 Minutes

Servings: 6

Ingredients:

- Two tablespoons olive oil
- 1 cup sliced fresh mushrooms
- 1 cup shredded spinach
- Six bacon slices, cooked and chopped
- Ten large eggs, beaten

- ½ cup crumbled goat cheese
- Sea salt
- Freshly ground black pepper

Directions:

1. Preheat the oven to 350 F.
2. Place an ovenproof frypan over medium-high heat and add the olive oil.
3. Cook the mushrooms until lightly browned, about 3 minutes.
4. Add the spinach and bacon and sauté until the greens are wilted, about 1 minute.
5. Add the eggs and cook, lifting the frittata's edges with a spatula so uncooked egg flow underneath, for 3 to 4 minutes.
6. Sprinkling the top with the crumbled goat cheese and season lightly with salt and pepper.
7. Bake until set and lightly browned, about 15 minutes.
8. Remove the frittata from the oven, and let it stand for 5 minutes.
9. Cut into six wedges and serve immediately.

Nutrition:

Calories: 316

Fat: 27g

Protein: 16g

Carbs: 1g

Fiber: 0g

Breakfast Bake

Preparation Time: 10 Minutes

Cooking Time: 50 Minutes

Servings: 8

Ingredients:

- One tablespoon olive oil, plus extra for greasing the casserole dish
- 1-pound preservative-free or homemade sausage
- Eight large eggs
- 2 cups cooked spaghetti squash
- One tablespoon chopped fresh oregano
- Sea salt
- Freshly ground black pepper
- ½ cup shredded Cheddar cheese

Directions:

1. Preheat the oven to 375 F.
2. Lightly grease a 9-by-13-inch casserole dish with olive oil and set aside.
3. Place an ovenproof skillet over medium-high heat, then add the olive oil.
4. Brown the sausage until cooked through, about 5 minutes. While the sausage is cooking, whisk together the eggs, squash, and oregano in a medium bowl. Season lightly with salt and pepper and set aside.
5. Add the cooked sausage to the egg mixture, stir until just combined, and pour it into the cooking pot.

6. Sprinkle with cheese and cover the casserole loosely with aluminum foil.

7. Bake the casserole for 30 minutes, remove the foil and bake for an additional 15 minutes.

8. Let the casserole stand for 10 minutes before serving.

Nutrition:

Calories: 303

Fat: 24g

Protein: 17g

Carbs: 4g

Fiber: 1g

Avocado and Eggs

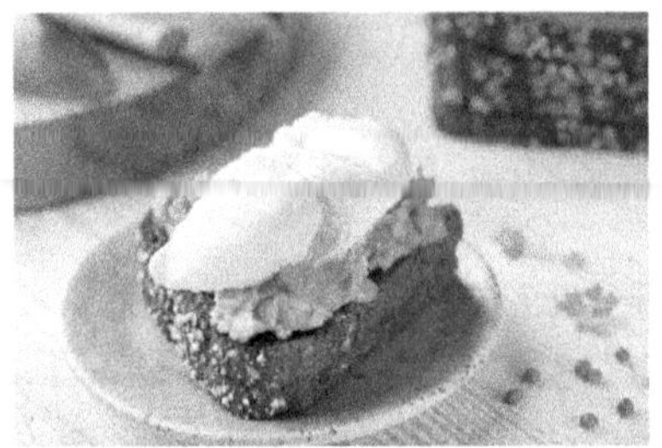

Preparation Time: 10 Minutes

Cooking Time: 20 Minutes

Servings: 4

Ingredients:

- Two avocados, peeled, halved lengthwise, and pitted
- Four large eggs
- 1 (4-ounce) chicken breast, cooked and shredded
- ¼ cup Cheddar cheese
- Sea salt
- Freshly ground black pepper

Directions:

1. Preheat the oven to 425 F.
2. Take a spoon and hollow each side of the avocado halves until the hole is about twice the original size.
3. Place the avocado halves in an 8-by-8-inch baking dish, hollow side up.
4. Crack an egg into each hollow and divide the shredded chicken between each avocado half. Sprinkle the cheese on top of each and season lightly with salt and pepper.
5. Bake the avocados until the eggs are cooked through, about 15 to 20 minutes.
6. Serve immediately.

Nutrition:

Calories: 324

Fat: 25g

Protein: 19g

Carbs: 8g

Fiber: 5g

Morning Buzz Iced Coffee

Preparation Time: 10 Minutes

Cooking Time: 0 Minutes

Servings: 1

Ingredients:

- 1 cup freshly brewed strong black coffee, cooled slightly
- One tablespoon extra-virgin olive oil
- One tablespoon half-and-half or heavy cream (optional)

- One teaspoon MCT oil (optional)
- 1/8 teaspoon almond extract
- 1/8 teaspoon ground cinnamon

Directions:

1. Pour the slightly cooled coffee into a blender or large glass (if using an immersion blender).
2. Add the olive oil, half-and-half (if using), MCT oil (if using), almond extract, and cinnamon.
3. Blend well until smooth and creamy. Drink warm and enjoy.

Nutrition:

Calories: 128

Total Fat: 14g

Total Carbs: 0g

Protein: 0g

Frittata

Preparation Time: 10 Minutes

Cooking Time: 15 Minutes

Servings: 2

Ingredients:

- Four large eggs
- Two tablespoons fresh chopped herbs, such as rosemary, thyme, oregano, basil, or one teaspoon dried herbs
- ¼ teaspoon salt
- Freshly ground black pepper
- Four tablespoons extra-virgin olive oil, divided
- 1 cup fresh spinach, arugula, kale, or other leafy greens
- 4 ounces quartered artichoke hearts, rinsed, drained, and thoroughly dried

- Eight cherry tomatoes halved
- ½ cup crumbled soft goat cheese

Directions:

1. Preheat the oven to broil on low.
2. In a small bowl, blend the eggs, herbs, salt, and pepper and whisk well with a fork. Set aside.
3. In a 4- to 5-inch oven-safe skillet or omelet pan, heat two tablespoons of olive oil over medium heat. Add the spinach, artichoke hearts, cherry tomatoes, and sauté until just wilted 1 to 2 minutes.
4. Pour in the egg mixture, then cook undisturbed over medium heat for 3 to 4 minutes, until the eggs begin to set on the bottom.
5. Sprinkle the goat cheese across the top of the egg mixture and transfer the skillet to the oven.
6. Broil for 4 to 5 minutes, or until the frittata is firm in the center and golden brown on top.
7. Take away from the oven and run a rubber spatula around the edge to loosen the sides. Invert onto a large plate or cutting board and slice in half. Serve warm and drizzled with the remaining two tablespoons of olive oil.

Nutrition:

Calories: 527 Total Fat: 47g

Total Carbs: 10g

Fiber: 3g Protein: 21g

Green Goddess Smoothie

Preparation Time: 5 Minutes

Cooking Time: 0 Minutes

Servings: 1

Ingredients:

- One small, very ripe avocado, peeled and pitted
- 1 cup almond milk or water, plus more as needed
- 1 cup tender baby spinach leaves, stems removed
- ½ medium cucumber, peeled and seeded
- One tablespoon extra-virgin olive oil or avocado oil
- 8 to 10 fresh mint leaves, stems removed
- Juice of 1 lime (about 1 to 2 tablespoons)

Directions:

1. In a blender or a large wide-mouth jar, combine the avocado, almond milk, spinach, cucumber, olive oil, mint, and lime juice and blend until smooth and creamy, adding more almond milk or water to achieve your desired consistency.

Nutrition:

Calories: 330

Total Fat: 30g

Total Carbs: 19g

Fiber: 9g

Protein: 4g

Blueberry Power Smoothie

Preparation Time: 5 Minutes

Cooking Time: 0 Minutes

Servings: 1

Ingredients:

- 1 cup unsweetened almond milk
- ¼ cup frozen blueberries
- Two tablespoons unsweetened almond butter
- One tablespoon ground flaxseed or chia seeds
- One tablespoon extra-virgin olive oil or avocado oil
- 1 to 2 teaspoons stevia or monk fruit extract (optional)
- ½ teaspoon vanilla extract
- ¼ teaspoon ground cinnamon

Directions:

1. In a blender or a large wide-mouth jar, mix the almond milk, blueberries, almond butter, flaxseed, olive oil, stevia (if using), vanilla, and cinnamon.
2. Blend until even and creamy, adding more almond milk to achieve your desired consistency.

Nutrition:

Calories: 460

Total Fat: 40g

Total Carbs: 20g

Fiber: 10g

Protein: 9g

Spiced Orange-Pistachio Smoothie

Preparation Time: 5 Minutes

Cooking Time: 0 Minutes

Servings: 1

Ingredients:

- ½ cup plain whole-milk Greek yogurt
- ½ cup unsweetened almond milk
- Juice of 1 clementine or ½ orange
- One tablespoon extra-virgin olive oil or MCT oil
- One tablespoon shelled pistachio, coarsely chopped
- 1 to 2 teaspoons monk fruit extract or stevia (optional)
- ¼ to ½ teaspoon ground allspice or unsweetened pumpkin pie spice
- ¼ teaspoon ground cinnamon
- ¼ teaspoon vanilla extract

Directions:

1. In a blender or a large wide-mouth jar, if using an immersion blender, combine the yogurt, ½ cup almond milk, clementine zest and juice, olive oil, pistachios, monk fruit extract (if using), allspice, cinnamon, and vanilla.
2. Blend until smooth and soft, adding more almond milk to achieve your desired consistency.

Nutrition:

Calories: 264

Total Fat: 22g

Total Carbs: 12g

Fiber: 2g

Protein: 6g

Florentine Breakfast Sandwich

Preparation Time: 10 Minutes

Cooking Time: 5 Minutes

Servings: 1

Ingredients:

- One teaspoon extra-virgin olive oil
- One large egg
- ¼ teaspoon salt
- ¼ teaspoon freshly ground black pepper
- 1 Versatile Sandwich Round

- One tablespoon jarred pesto
- ¼ ripe avocado, mashed
- 1 (¼-inch) thick tomato slice
- 1 (1-ounce) slice fresh mozzarella

Directions:

1. In a small fry pan, heat the olive oil over high heat. When the oil is very hot, crack the egg into the skillet and reduce the medium's heat. Sprinkle the top of the egg with salt and pepper and let it cook for 2 minutes, or until set on bottom.

2. Using a spatula, turn over the egg to cook on the other side to the desired level of doneness (1 to 2

minutes for a runnier yolk, 2 to 3 minutes for a harder yolk). Take away the egg from the pan and keep warm.

3. Cut the sandwich round in half horizontally and toast, if desired.

4. To assemble the sandwich, spread the pesto on a toasted bread half. Top with mashed avocado, the tomato slice, mozzarella, and the cooked egg. Top with the other bread half and eat warm.

Nutrition:

Calories: 548

Total Fat: 48g

Total Carbs: 8g

Fiber: 3g

Protein: 21g

Avocado Toast

Preparation Time: 5 Minutes

Cooking Time: 5 Minutes

Servings: 2

Ingredients:

- Two tablespoons ground flaxseed
- ½ teaspoon baking powder
- Two large eggs
- One teaspoon salt, plus more for serving
- ½ teaspoon freshly ground black pepper
- ½ teaspoon garlic powder, sesame seed, caraway seed, or other dried herbs (optional)
- Three tablespoons extra-virgin olive oil, divided
- One medium ripe avocado, peeled, pitted, and sliced

- Two tablespoons chopped ripe tomato or salsa

Directions:

1. In a small bowl, blend the flaxseed and baking powder, breaking up any lumps in the baking powder. Add the eggs, pepper, salt, and garlic powder (if using) and whisk well. Let sit for 2 minutes.

2. In a small nonstick skillet, heat one tablespoon olive oil over medium heat. Decant the egg mixture into the skillet and let cook undisturbed until the egg begins to set on the bottom, 2 to 3 minutes.

3. By means of a rubber spatula, scrape down the sides to allow uncooked egg to reach the bottom. Cook another 2 to 3 minutes.

4. Once almost set, flip like a pancake and allow the top to cook thoroughly for another 1 to 2 minutes.

5. Take away from the pan and allow to cool slightly. Slice into two pieces.

6. Top each "toast" with avocado slices, additional salt and pepper, chopped tomato, and drizzle with the remaining two tablespoons olive oil.

Nutrition:

Calories: 287 Total Fat: 25g

Total Carbs: 10g

Protein: 9g

Baklava Hot Porridge

Preparation Time: 5 Minutes

Cooking Time: 5 Minutes

Servings: 2

Ingredients:

- 2 cups Riced Cauliflower
- ¾ cup unsweetened almond, flax, or hemp milk
- Four tablespoons extra-virgin olive oil, divided
- Two teaspoons grated fresh orange peel (from ½ orange)
- ½ teaspoon ground cinnamon
- ½ teaspoon almond extract or vanilla extract
- 1/8 teaspoon salt
- Four tablespoons chopped walnuts, divided
- 1 to 2 teaspoons liquid stevia, monk fruit, or another sweetener of choice (optional)

Directions:

1. In a medium saucepan, combine the riced cauliflower, almond milk, two tablespoons olive oil, grated orange peel, cinnamon, almond extract, and salt. Stir to combine and boil over medium-high heat, stirring constantly.
2. Remove from heat and stir in 2 tablespoons chopped walnuts and sweetener (if using). Stir to combine.
3. Divide into bowls, topping each with one tablespoon of chopped walnuts and one

tablespoon of the remaining olive oil.

Nutrition:

Calories: 382

Total Fat: 38g

Total Carbs: 11g

Protein: 5g

Lemon–Olive Oil Breakfast Cakes with Berry Syrup

Preparation Time: 5 Minutes

Cooking Time: 10 Minutes

Servings: 4

Ingredients:

For the Pancakes

- 1 cup almond flour
- One teaspoon baking powder
- ¼ teaspoon salt

- Six tablespoon extra-virgin olive oil, divided
- Two large eggs
- Zest and juice of 1 lemon
- ½ teaspoon almond or vanilla extract

For the Berry Sauce

- 1 cup of frozen mixed berries
- One tablespoon water or lemon juice, plus more if needed
- ½ teaspoon vanilla extract

Directions:

To Make the Pancakes

1. In a large bowl, blend the almond flour, baking powder, salt, and whisk to break up any clumps.
2. Add the four tablespoons olive oil,

eggs, lemon zest and juice, and almond extract and whisk to combine well.

3. In a large skillet, heat one tablespoon of olive oil and spoon about two tablespoons of batter for each of 4 pancakes. Cook until bubbles begin to form, 4 to 5 minutes, and flip. Cook another 2 to 3 minutes on the second side. Repeat with the remaining one tablespoon olive oil and batter.

To Make the Berry Sauce

4. In a small saucepan, heat the frozen berries, water, and vanilla extract over medium-high for 3 to 4 minutes, until bubbly, adding more water if the mixture is too thick. By means of the back of a spoon, mash the berries and whisk until smooth.

Nutrition:

Calories: 275

Total Fat: 26g

Total Carbs: 8g

Protein: 4g

Greek Yogurt Parfait

Preparation Time: 5 Minutes

Cooking Time: 0 Minutes

Servings: 1

Ingredients:

- ½ cup plain whole-milk Greek yogurt
- Two tablespoons heavy whipping cream

- ¼ cup frozen berries, thawed with juices
- ½ teaspoon vanilla or almond extract (optional)
- ¼ teaspoon ground cinnamon (optional)
- One tablespoon ground flaxseed
- Two tablespoons chopped nuts (walnuts or pecans)

Directions:

1. In a small bowl or glass, blend the yogurt, heavy whipping cream, thawed berries in their juice, vanilla or almond extract (if using), cinnamon (if using), flaxseed, and stir well until smooth. Top with chopped nuts and enjoy.

Nutrition:

Calories: 267

Total Fat: 19g

Total Carbs: 12g

Protein: 12g

Egg Baked in Avocado

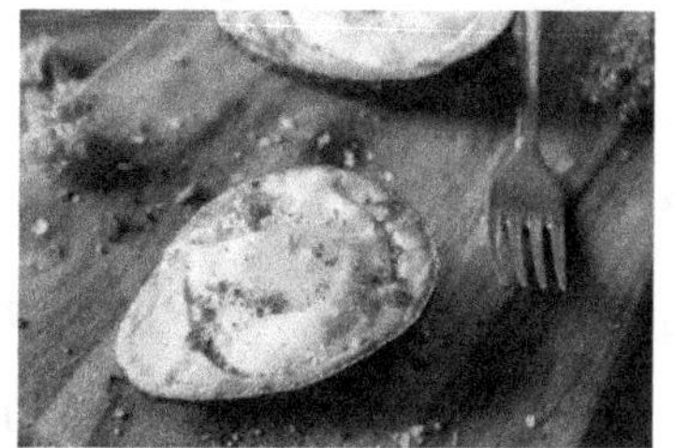

Preparation Time: 5 Minutes

Cooking Time: 15 Minutes

Servings: 2

Ingredients:

- One large ripe avocado
- Two large eggs
- Salt
- Freshly ground black pepper

- Four tablespoons jarred pesto, for serving
- Two tablespoons chopped tomato, for serving
- Two tablespoons crumbled feta, for serving (optional)

Directions:

1. Preheat the oven to 425 F.
2. Cut the avocado in and take away the pit. Scoop out about 1 to 2 tablespoons from each half to create a hole large enough to fit an egg. Place the avocado halves on a baking sheet, cut-side up.
3. Crack one egg in each avocado half and season with pepper and salt.
4. Bake and wait for the eggs are set and cooked to the wanted level of doneness, 10 to 15 minutes.
5. Remove from oven and top each avocado with two tablespoons pesto, one tablespoon chopped tomato, and one tablespoon crumbled feta (if using).

Nutrition:

Calories: 302 Total Fat: 26g

Total Carbs: 10g

Protein: 8g

Cheese Crepes

Preparation Time: 15 Minutes

Cooking Time: 20 Minutes

Servings: 5

Ingredients:

- 6 ounces cream cheese

- 1/3 cup Parmesan cheese
- Six large organic eggs
- One teaspoon granulated erythritol
- 1½ tablespoon coconut flour
- 1/8 teaspoon xanthan gum
- Two tablespoons unsalted butter

Directions:

1. Pulse the cream cheese, Parmesan cheese, eggs, and erythritol using a blender.
2. Place the coconut flour and xanthan gum and pulse again.
3. Now, pulse at medium speed. Transfer and put aside within 5 minutes.
4. Melt butter over medium-low heat.
5. Place one portion of the mixture and tilt the pan to spread into a thin layer.
6. Cook within 1½ minutes.
7. Flip the crepe and cook within 15-20 seconds more. Serve.

Nutrition:

Calories 297

Net Carbs 1.9 g

Total Fat 25.1 g

Cholesterol 281 mg

Total Carbs 3.5 g

Protein 13.7 g

Ricotta Pancakes

Preparation Time: 10 Minutes

Cooking Time: 20 Minutes

Servings: 4

Ingredients:

- Four organic eggs
- ½ cup ricotta cheese
- ¼ cup of vanilla whey protein powder
- ½ teaspoon organic baking powder
- Salt
- ½ teaspoon liquid stevia
- Two tablespoons unsalted butter

Directions:

1. Pulse all the fixing in the blender.
2. Warm-up butter over medium heat.
3. Put the batter and spread it evenly. Cook within 2 minutes.
4. Flip and cook again within 1–2 minutes. Serve.

Nutrition:

Calories 184 Net Carbs 2.7 g

Total Fat 12.9 g

Total Carbs 2.7 g Protein 14.6 g

Yogurt Waffles

Preparation Time: 15 Minutes

Cooking Time: 25 Minutes

Servings: 5

Ingredients:

- ½ cup golden flax seeds meal

- ½ cup plus three tablespoons almond flour
- 1-1½ tablespoons granulated erythritol
- One tablespoon of vanilla whey protein powder
- ¼ teaspoon baking soda
- ½ teaspoon organic baking powder
- ¼ teaspoon xanthan gum
- Salt
- One large organic egg
- One organic egg
- Two tablespoons unsweetened almond milk
- 1½ tablespoons unsalted butter
- 3 ounces plain Greek yogurt

Directions:

1. Preheat the waffle iron, then grease it.
2. Mix add the flour, erythritol, protein powder, baking soda, baking powder, xanthan gum, and salt.
3. Beat the egg white until stiff peaks. In a third bowl, add two egg yolks, whole egg, almond milk, butter, yogurt, and beat.
4. Put egg mixture into the bowl of the flour mixture and mix.
5. Gently fold in the beaten egg whites. Place ¼ cup of the mixture into preheated waffle iron and cook for about 4–5 minutes. Serve.

Nutrition:

Calories 250 Net Carbs 3.2 g

Total Fat 18 7 g Protein 8 4 g

Broccoli Muffins

Preparation Time: 15 Minutes

Cooking Time: 20 Minutes

Servings: 6

Ingredients:

- Two tablespoons unsalted butter
- Six large organic eggs
- ½ cup heavy whipping cream
- ½ cup Parmesan cheese
- Salt & ground black pepper
- 1¼ cups broccoli
- Two tablespoons parsley
- ½ cup Swiss cheese

Directions:

1. Warm-up oven to 350°F, then grease a 12-cup muffin tin.
2. Mix the eggs, cream, Parmesan cheese, salt, and black pepper.
3. Divide the broccoli and parsley in the muffin cup.
4. Top with the egg mixture, with Swiss cheese.
5. Bake within 20 minutes. Cool for about 5 minutes. Serve.

Nutrition:

Calories 231 Net Carbs 2 g

Total Fat 18.1 g

Cholesterol 228 mg

Protein 13.5 g

Pumpkin Bread

Preparation Time: 15 Minutes

Cooking Time: 60 Minutes

Servings: 16

Ingredients:

- 1 2/3 cups almond flour
- 1½ teaspoons organic baking powder
- ½ teaspoon pumpkin pie spice
- ½ teaspoon cinnamon
- ½ teaspoon cloves
- ½ teaspoon salt
- 8 ounces cream cheese
- Six organic eggs
- One tablespoon coconut flour
- 1 cup powdered erythritol
- One teaspoon stevia powder
- One teaspoon organic lemon extract
- 1 cup pumpkin puree
- ½ cup of coconut oil

Directions:

1. Warm-up oven to 325°F. Grease 2 bread loaf pans.
2. Mix the almond flour, baking powder, spices, and salt in a small bowl.
3. In a second bowl, add the cream cheese, one egg, coconut flour, ¼ cup of erythritol, and ¼ teaspoon of the stevia, and beat.
4. In a third bowl, add the pumpkin puree, oil, five eggs, ¾ cup of the

erythritol, and ¾ teaspoon of the stevia and mix.

5. Mix the pumpkin mixture into the bowl of the flour mixture.

6. Place about ¼ of the pumpkin mixture into each loaf pan.

7. Top each pan with the cream cheese mixture, plus the rest pumpkin mixture.

8. Bake within 50–60 minutes. Cold within 10 minutes. Slice and serve.

Nutrition:

Calories 216

Net Carbs 2.5 g

Total Fat 19.8 g

Cholesterol 77 mg

Protein 3.4 g

Eggs in Avocado Cups

Preparation Time: 10 Minutes

Cooking Time: 20 Minutes

Servings: 4

Ingredients:

- Two avocados
- Four organic eggs
- Salt
- Ground black pepper
- Four tablespoons cheddar cheese
- Two cooked bacon
- One tablespoon scallion green

Directions:

1. Warm-up oven to 400°F. Remove two tablespoons of flesh from the avocado.

2. Place avocado halves into a small baking dish.

3. Crack an egg in each avocado half and sprinkle with salt plus black pepper.

4. Top each egg with cheddar cheese evenly.

5. Bake within 20 minutes. Serve with bacon and chives.

Nutrition:

Calories 343 Net Carbs 2.2 g

Total Fat 29.1 g

Cholesterol 186 mg

Protein 13.8 g

Cheddar Scramble

Preparation Time: 10 Minutes

Cooking Time: 8 Minutes

Servings: 6

Ingredients:

- Two tablespoons olive oil

- One small yellow onion

- 12 large organic eggs

- Salt and ground black pepper

- 4 ounces cheddar cheese

Directions:

1. Warm-up oil over medium heat.

2. Sauté the onion within 4–5 minutes.

3. Add the eggs, salt, and black pepper and cook within 3 minutes.

4. Remove then stir in the cheese. Serve.

Nutrition:

Calories 264 Net Carbs 1.8 g

Total Fat 20.9 g

Cholesterol 392 mg

Protein 17.4 g

Bacon Omelet

Preparation Time: 10 Minutes

Cooking Time: 15 Minutes

Servings: 2

Ingredients:

- Four organic eggs
- One tablespoon chive
- Salt
- ground black pepper
- Four bacon slices
- One tablespoon unsalted butter
- 2 ounces cheddar cheese

Directions:

1. Beat the eggs, chives, salt, and black pepper in a bowl.
2. Warm-up a pan over medium-high heat then cooks the bacon slices within 8–10 minutes.
3. Chop the bacon slices. Melt butter and cook the egg mixture within 2 minutes.
4. Flip the omelet and top with chopped bacon. Cook within 1–2 minutes.
5. Remove then put the cheese in the center of the omelet. Serve.

Nutrition:

Calories 427

Net Carbs 1.2 g

Total Fat 28.2 g

Cholesterol 469 mg

Protein 29.1 g

Green Veggies Quiche

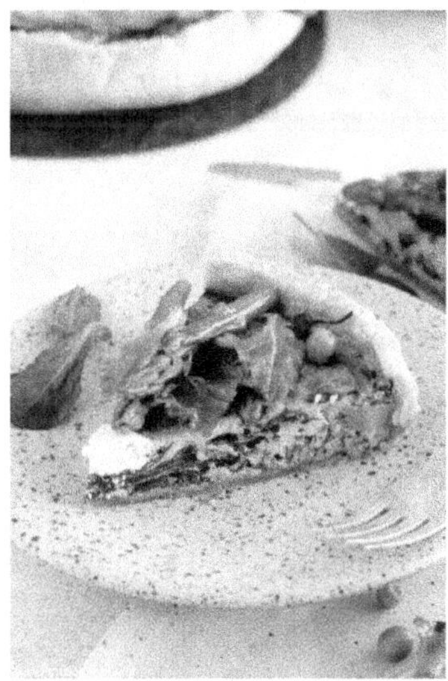

Preparation Time: 20 Minutes

Cooking Time: 20 Minutes

Servings: 4

Ingredients:

- Six organic eggs
- ½ cup unsweetened almond milk
- Salt and ground black pepper
- 2 cups baby spinach
- ½ cup green bell pepper
- One scallion
- ¼ cup cilantro
- One tablespoon chive,
- Three tablespoons mozzarella cheese

Directions:

1. Warm-up oven to 400°F.
2. Grease a pie dish. Beat eggs, almond milk, salt, and black pepper. Set aside.
3. In another bowl, add the vegetables and herbs, then mix.
4. Place the veggie mixture and top with the egg mixture in the pie dish.
5. Bake within 20 minutes. Remove then sprinkle with the Parmesan cheese.

6. Slice and serve.

Nutrition:

Calories 176 Net Carbs 4.1 g

Total Fat 10.9 g

Cholesterol 257 mg

Protein 15.4 g

Chicken & Asparagus Frittata

Preparation Time: 15 Minutes

Cooking Time: 12 Minutes

Servings: 4

Ingredients:

- ½ cup grass-fed chicken breast
- 1/3 cup Parmesan cheese
- Six organic eggs
- Salt
- ground black pepper
- 1/3 cup boiled asparagus
- ¼ cup cherry tomatoes
- ¼ cup mozzarella cheese

Directions:

1. Warm-up broiler of the oven, then mix Parmesan cheese, eggs, salt, and black pepper in a bowl.
2. Melt butter, then cook the chicken and asparagus within 2–3 minutes.
3. Add the egg mixture and tomatoes and mix. Cook within 4–5 minutes.
4. Remove then sprinkle with the Parmesan cheese.
5. Transfer the wok under the broiler and broil

within 3–4 minutes. Slice and serve.

Nutrition:

Calories 158 Net Carbs 1.3 g

Total Fat 9.3 g

Cholesterol 265 mg

Southwest Scrambled Egg Bites

Preparation Time: 10 Minutes

Cooking Time: 23 Minutes

Servings: 4

Ingredients:

- Five eggs
- 1/2 teaspoon hot pepper sauce
- 1/3 cup tomatoes
- Three tablespoons green chilies
- One teaspoon black pepper
- 1/2 teaspoon salt
- Two tablespoons nondairy milk

Directions:

1. Mix both the eggs and milk in a large cup.
2. Add the hot sauce, pepper, and salt.
3. Put a small diced chilies and diced tomatoes in silicone cups. Fill each with 3/4 full with the egg mixture.
4. Put the trivet in the pot and pour 1 cup water. Put the mold on the trivet.
5. Set too high for 8 minutes. Cooldown before serving.

Nutrition:

Calories: 106

Carbs: 2g Protein: 7.5g

Fats: 7.4g

Bacon Egg Bites

Preparation Time: 10 Minutes

Cooking Time: 22 Minutes

Servings: 9

Ingredients:

- 1 cup cheese
- 1/2 green pepper
- 1/2 cup cottage cheese
- Four slices of bacon
- Pepper
- Salt
- 1 cup red onion
- 1 cup of water
- 1/4 cup whip cream
- 1/4 cup egg whites
- Four eggs

Directions:

1. Blend egg whites, eggs, cream, cheese (cottage), shredded cheese, pepper, and salt within 30 to 45 seconds in a blender.
2. Put the egg mixture into mini muffin cups. Top each with bacon, peppers, and onion.
3. Cover the muffin cups tightly with foil. Place the trivet in the pot and pour 1 cup water.
4. Put the cups on the trivet. Set to steam for 12 minutes. Cooldown before serving.

Nutrition:

Calories: 124

Carbs: 3g

Protein: 9g

Fats: 8

Omelet Bites

Preparation Time: 5 Minutes

Cooking Time: 8 Minutes

Servings: 3

Ingredients:

- One handful mushrooms
- Green onion
- Green peppers
- 1/8 teaspoon hot sauce
- Pepper, salt, mustard, garlic powder
- 1/2 cup cheese cheddar
- 1/2 cup cheese cottage
- Two deli ham slices
- Four eggs

Directions:

1. Whisk eggs, then the cheddar and cottage. Put the ham, veggies, and seasonings; mix.
2. Pour the mixture into greased silicone molds. Put the trivet with the molds in the pot, then fill with 2 cups water.
3. Steam for about 8 minutes. Transfer, cooldown before serving.

Nutrition: Calories: 260

Carbs: 6g Protein: 22g Fats: 16g

Cheddar & Bacon Egg Bites

Preparation Time: 10 Minutes

Cooking Time: 8 Minutes

Servings: 7

Ingredients:

- 1 cup sharp cheddar cheese

- One tablespoon parsley flake
- Four eggs
- Four tablespoons cream
- Hot sauce
- 1 cup of water
- 1/2 cup cheese
- Four slices of bacon

Directions:

1. Blend the cream, cheddar, cottage, and egg in the blender; 30 seconds.
2. Stir in the parsley—grease silicone egg bite molds.
3. Divide the crumbled bacon between them. Put the egg batter into each cup.
4. With a piece of foil, cover each mold. Place the trivet with the molds in the pot, then fill with 1 cup water.
5. Steam for 8 minutes. Remove, let rest for 5 minutes. Serve, sprinkled with black pepper, and optional hot sauce.

Nutrition:

Calories: 167 Fats: 11.7g

Carbs: 1.5g Protein: 13.5g

Avocado Pico Egg Bites

Preparation Time: 15 Minutes

Cooking Time: 10 Minutes

Servings: 7

Ingredients:

Egg bites:

- 1/ cup cheese cottage
- 1/2 cup cheese Mexican blend

- 1/4 cup cream heavy cream
- 1/4 teaspoon chili powder
- 1/4 teaspoon cumin
- 1/4 teaspoon garlic powder
- Four eggs
- Pepper
- Salt

Pico de Gallo:

- One avocado
- One jalapeno
- 1/2 teaspoon salt
- 1/4 onion
- Two tablespoons cilantro
- Two teaspoons lime juice
- 4 Roma tomatoes

Directions:

1. Mix all of the Pico de Gallo fixing except for the avocado. Gently fold in the avocado.
2. Blend all the egg bites ingredients in a blender. Spoon one tablespoon of Pico de Gallo into each egg bite silicone mold.
3. Place the trivet in the pot, then fill with 1 cup water. Put the molds in the trivet. Set to high within 10 minutes.
4. Remove. Serve topped with cheese and Pico de Gallo.

Nutrition:

Calories: 118

Carbs: 1g

Protein: 7g

Fats: 9g

Keto Mushroom Omelet

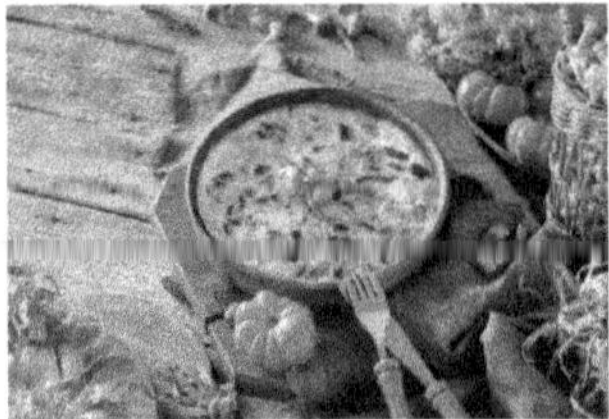

Preparation Time: 5 Minutes

Cooking Time: 12 Minutes

Servings: 2

Ingredients:

- Three large egg
- Two tablespoons of butter
- Eighty gram of cremini mushroom,
- sliced
- 1-ounce cheddar cheese, shredded
- One-quarter of medium red onion, diced
- Salt and pepper to taste

Directions:

1. Ingredients for preparation: cut the cheese, dice the mushrooms and chop the onion.

2. Crack the eggs in a bowl and apply a touch of salt and pepper to taste. Whisk with a fork until it is mildly frothy and combined.

3. In a frying pan, heat the fat. Apply to the pan the diced red onion and sliced mushrooms. Season to taste, then fry, stirring regularly, until the mushrooms are tender. Pour on top of the egg mixture, meaning it gets past the onions and mushrooms.

4. Sprinkle the cheddar cheese over the top of the omelet.

5. Move under the omelet carefully with a spatula and fold it in half.

6. Remove from the skillet and eat warm if the omelet on the bottom is golden brown.

Nutrition:

Calories 586

Fat 48.2g

Net Carbs 6.9g

Protein 29.7g

Crepes Keto

Preparation Time: 5 Minutes

Cooking Time: 15 Minutes

Servings: 5

Ingredients:

- Four large eggs

- Half cup of almond flour

- Four ounces of cream cheese softened

- Two tablespoons of stevia erythritol blend 23

- One-quarter cup of unsweetened almond milk

Directions:

1. Gather all of the ingredients and wash them.

2. To a blender, add all ingredients, then pump until smooth and well mixed. Let them relax for a couple of minutes.

3. Spray just enough cooking spray into a non-stick pan over medium-low heat to coat the bottom of the pan. Add in 1-2

tablespoons of butter until warm.

4. To disperse the batter into a thin sheet, stir the pan.

5. Cook the crepe until the sides are very hardened, and a spatula may remove the rim. On the other side, flip and cook until it achieves a light golden-brown color.

6. Repeat with all the batter in this process. Fill or top with any preferred fillers.

7. Serve it hot and appreciate it! For some added esthetic, feel free to add a few extra berries or powdered erythritol

Nutrition:

Calories 297

Fat 25.2g

Net Carbs 3.7g

Protein 12.6g

Keto Mushroom Sausage Skillet

Preparation Time: 5 Minutes

Cooking Time: 25 Minutes

Servings: 5

Ingredients:

- Sixteen ounces of cremini mushroom
- Sixteen ounces of pork sausage
- One cup of mozzarella cheese, grated
- Two tablespoons of olive oil
- Two medium green onions, for garnish

Directions:

1. Collect all ingredients and cook them.

2. To heat it, switch on the oven to broil.

3. Load half the olive oil onto a cast iron skillet and switch on medium heat on the stovetop.

4. Wash the mushrooms, dry them well with a paper towel, and cut them into strips.

5. Cook the sausages in the cast iron skillet on the stovetop over medium to high heat until they are golden and thoroughly fried. Remove the sausages from the pan until they are thoroughly cooked and arrange them on a cutting board.

6. Add the remaining olive oil to the skillet, add the mushrooms and cook until the mushrooms are golden brown.

7. Chop up the pork sausage on a cutting board while the mushrooms are frying, with a diagonal break.

8. Add the sliced pork sausage to the skillet and scatter with mozzarella cheese as soon as the mushrooms are thoroughly cooked. Place it on a grill inside the oven until the cheese begins to melt. Look closely at the microwave. The cheese melts quickly!

9. Remove and garnish with green onions from the oven.

Nutrition:

Calories 357 Fat 25g

Carbohydrates 4.5g

Protein 22g

Keto Benedict Eggs

Preparation Time: 5 Minutes

Cooking Time: 25 Minutes

Servings: 3

Ingredients:

- Hollandaise Sauce
- Three large egg yolks
- Three tablespoons of butter
- One teaspoon of lemon juice
- Salt and paprika, to taste
- Eggs Benedict
- Three servings 90-second keto mug bread Four large eggs
- Five-ounce Canadian bacon, about 4
- small slices
- One tablespoon of white vinegar
- Two teaspoons of butter
- One tablespoon of chives, chopped
- Salt, as needed

Directions:

1. Gather all of the ingredients and wash them. Prepare, slice, and set aside the 90-second keto mug bread.

2. Set a pot of water on the stove to boil (about 1-2 inches worth of water). Switch down to medium-low to simmer during heating.

3. Separate the egg yolks and put aside the whites for another recipe. In a metal bowl, beat the egg yolks until their shiny and deep purple. Apply the lemon juice and whisk again until mixed.

4. In the microwave or a pan, heat the butter.

Place the metal bowl over the pot like a double boiler until it is hot. As the egg yolk mixture heats up, slowly add the butter while whisking together to emulsify.

5. When the mixture comes together and thickens up, keep whisking away. As the eggs get scrambled, if they get too wet, ensure not to add too many heats to the mix. The mixture will cover the back of a spoon well until finished. You can slide your finger over it and see the indentation plainly from where you swipe if you plunge a spoon in.

6. With salt and paprika, season the hollandaise and put aside.

7. If required, you want between 3-4 inches of water to fill the water pot with more water. To get the water to boil, set the heat to medium-high again. Decrease the heat to steam because it is boiling, then apply salt and vinegar to the bath.

8. Crack an egg into a little dish or ramekin. Stir the boiling water in a pot using a spoon to create a water spout, then gently dump the egg into the water.

9. Try not to lose the egg when you want it to poach and keep together.

10. Allow the egg simmer for 2-3 minutes, after which take it out using a slotted spoon from the pan. Place the paper towels gently on a plate and repeat the procedure with the other eggs.

11. Fry the Canadian bacon in a different pan until slightly browned on both sides, or to your taste.

12. Toast the mug bread with butter if desired, or simply sprinkle butter over the top of each slice.

13. Assemble Benedict's eggs. On top of each other, put one slice of mug bread, Canadian bacon, and a poached egg. If needed, season the egg with salt and pepper. With the remainder of the mug bread, Canadian bacon, and eggs, repeat this process.

14. Finally, spoon the combination of Hollandaise over the top of the eggs. You should pour a small volume of water into it and stir together until it's spooned able again if the hollandaise has gotten too thick. Garnish with sliced chives and serve!

Nutrition:

calories 780

protein 53g

Fat 60.5g

Carbs 6.0g

Replacement Shake for Keto Meal

Preparation Time: 7 Minutes

Cooking Time: 0 Minutes

Servings: 1

Ingredients:

- Half cup of heavy cream
- Half medium of avocado
- Two tablespoons of almond butter
- Two tablespoons of golden flaxseed meal
- One cup of unsweetened almond milk from the carton
- Two tablespoons of cocoa powder
- Half teaspoon of cinnamon
- Fifteen drops of liquid stevia to taste
- One-quarter tablespoon of vanilla extract
- Eight whole ice cubes
- A pinch of salt to taste

Directions:

1. Pit and peel the avocado-keep your ingredients prepped.

2. In a blender, add all the ingredients, slowly process together until blended, then mix for 30-45 seconds until a smooth consistency emerges.

3. I propose that you apply half the sweetener to the shake, sample it, and change the sweetener according to your preference.

4. Pour out into a bottle if you have the right consistency and enjoy!

Nutrition:

Calories 449

Fats 42.0g

Carbohydrates 7.0g

Protein 9.0g

Keto Cauliflower Hash Browns

Preparation Time: 5 Minutes

Cooking Time: 35 Minutes

Servings: 3

Ingredients:

- sixteen ounces of cauliflower
- three large eggs
- half medium-sized onion
- one teaspoon of salt
- black pepper
- eight tablespoons of butter

Directions:

1. By means of either a grater or a food processor, grate the cauliflower and onion into tiny pieces.
2. In a cup, add the cauliflower and onion and add the eggs and seasoning. Mix well with each other and set aside for 5-10 minutes.
3. Melt enough butter to coat the pan's bottom thoroughly.
4. Apply scoops of cauliflower mixture to the butter and fry on either side for 4-5 minutes. As they will fall away, be careful not to turn until the sides are crispy. To help fry the hash browns, add additional butter to the pan as needed.

5. To help keep them warm, you can keep the finished cauliflower hash browns in foil if you cook in batches. Serve the hash browns with the butter from the pan until done.

Nutrition:

Calories 300 Fat 26.6g

Carbohydrates 3.12g

Protein 7.58g

Keto Crepes Dairy Free

Preparation Time: 5 Minutes

Cooking Time: 10 Minutes

Servings: 3

Ingredients:

- One-quarter cup of almond flour
- two tablespoons of coconut flour
- one-quarter teaspoon of salt
- four large eggs
- one-third cup of coconut milk, canned Dairy-Free Whipped Cream
- twelve ounces of overnight chilled coconut milk
- half cup of powdered form of erythritol blend
- three medium sliced strawberries

Directions:

1. Combine the almond flour, coconut flour, salt, and eggs and process until fluffy in a blender.
2. With a spatula, scrape the sides and add coconut milk at room temperature.

3. Blend until perfectly smooth.

4. To finish absorbing some excess material, let the batter rest for about five minutes.

5. Heat to medium with a non-stick skillet. In the skillet, add about two tablespoons plus a little more flour and tilt it softly from side to side until the flour stretches into a thin pancake. It's not an absolute calculation because your pan and how thin you like your crepe will depend on it.

6. Raise the edges softly after the sides are set and turn to cook on the other side for about 30 seconds. Place and repeat on a plate until the batter is out.

7. The cold coconut cream and sweetener beat until smooth by using a stand mixer's whisk fitting or handheld electric blender.

8. Cover crepes with whipped cream without dairy and incorporate new strawberries.

Nutrition:

Calories 699.4 Fats 66.84g

Carbs 10.4g Protein 22.44g

Eggs and Traditional Bacon

Preparation Time: 5 Minutes

Cooking Time: 25 Minutes

Servings: 5

Ingredients

- Eight large eggs

- five ounces of bacon, sliced.
- About 14 cherry tomatoes
- One-quarter cup of fresh parsley, chopped

Directions:

1. Fry the bacon slices until they are crunchy, over mcdium-high heat. Put aside the bacon but leave the pan with the bacon fat.
2. In the hot bacon fat, break the eggs open. Cook them as much as you want.
3. Season the salt and pepper with the eggs, then apply the bacon to the pan.
4. In the hot skillet, introduce your cherry tomatoes and toast for a couple of minutes.
5. Serve the eggs and bacon with the onions, next marinade mostly with parsley.

Nutrition:

Calories 332.39

Fats 23.15g

Carbohydrates 3.2g

Protein 25.23g

CHAPTER 6:

Snacks

Roasted Cauliflower with Prosciutto, Capers, and Almonds

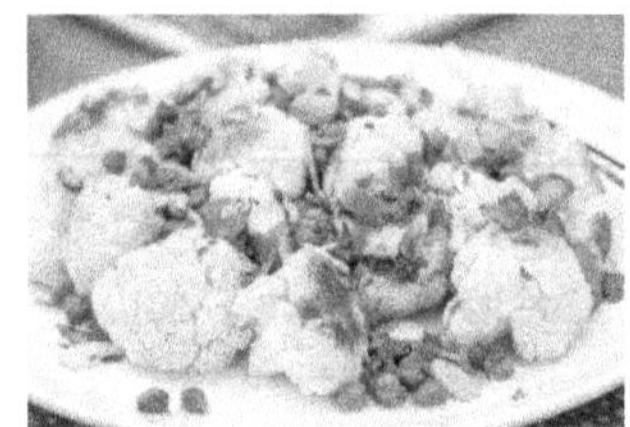

Preparation Time: 5 Minutes

Cooking Time: 25 Minutes

Servings: 2

Ingredients:

- 12 ounces cauliflower florets
- Two tablespoons leftover bacon grease or olive oil
- Pink Himalayan salt
- Freshly ground black pepper
- 2 ounces sliced prosciutto, torn into small pieces
- ¼ cup slivered almonds
- Two tablespoons capers
- Two tablespoons grated Parmesan cheese

Directions:

1. Preheat the oven to 400 F. Line a baking pan with a silicone baking mat or parchment paper.
2. Put the cauliflower florets in the prepared baking pan with the bacon grease and season with pink

Himalayan salt and pepper. Or if you are using olive oil instead, drizzle the cauliflower with olive oil and season with pink Himalayan salt and pepper.

3. Roast the cauliflower for 15 minutes.

4. Stir the cauliflower so all sides are coated with the bacon grease.

5. Distribute the prosciutto pieces in the pan. Then add the slivered almonds and capers. Stir to combine. Sprinkle the Parmesan cheese on top, and roast for 10 minutes more.

6. Divide between two plates, using a slotted spoon, so you don't get excess grease in the plates, and serve.

Nutrition:

Calories: 288

Total Fat: 24g

Carbs: 7g

Fiber: 3g

Protein: 14g

Buttery Slow-Cooker Mushrooms

Preparation Time: 10 Minutes

Cooking Time: 4 Hours

Servings: 2

Ingredients:

- Six tablespoons butter
- One tablespoon packaged dry ranch dressing mix
- 8 ounces fresh cremini mushrooms
- Two tablespoons grated Parmesan cheese

- One tablespoon chopped fresh flat-leaf Italian parsley

Directions:

1. With the crock insert in place, preheat the slow cooker to low.

2. Put the butter and the dry ranch dressing in the bottom of the slow cooker, and allow the butter to melt. Stir to blend the dressing mix and butter.

3. Add the mushrooms to the slow cooker, and stir to coat with the butter-dressing mixture. Sprinkle the top with the Parmesan cheese.

4. Close its lid and cook on low for 4 hours.

5. Use a slotted spoon to transfer the mushrooms to a serving dish. Top with the chopped parsley and serve.

Nutrition:

Calories: 351

Total Fat: 36g

Carbs: 5g

Fiber: 1g

Protein: 6g

Baked Zucchini Gratin

Preparation Time: 10 Minutes

Cooking Time: 25 Minutes

Servings: 2

Ingredients:

- One large zucchini, cut into ¼-inch-thick slices
- Pink Himalayan salt
- 1-ounce Brie cheese, rind trimmed off
- One tablespoon butter

- Freshly ground black pepper
- 1/3 cup shredded Gruyère cheese
- ¼ cup crushed pork rinds

Directions:

1. Salt the zucchini slices and put them in a colander in the sink for 45 minutes; the zucchini will shed much of their water.
2. Preheat the oven to 400 F.
3. When the zucchini has been "weeping" for about 30 minutes, in a small saucepan over medium-low heat, heat the Brie and butter, occasionally stirring, until the cheese has melted and the mixture is thoroughly combined, about 2 minutes.
4. Arrange the zucchini in an 8-inch baking dish, so the zucchini slices overlap a bit—season with pepper.
5. Pour the Brie mixture over the zucchini, and top with the shredded Gruyère cheese.
6. Sprinkle the crushed pork rinds over the top.
7. Bake for about 25 minutes, until the dish is bubbling and the top is nicely browned, and serve.

Nutrition:

Calories: 355

Total Fat: 25g

Carbs: 5g

Fiber: 2g

Protein: 28g

Roasted Radishes with Brown Butter Sauce

Preparation Time: 10 Minutes

Cooking Time: 15 Minutes

Servings: 2

Ingredients:

- 2 cups halved radishes
- One tablespoon olive oil
- Pink Himalayan salt
- Freshly ground black pepper
- Two tablespoons butter
- One tablespoon chopped fresh flat-leaf Italian parsley

Directions:

1. Preheat the oven to 450 F.
2. In a medium bowl, toss the radishes in the olive oil and season with pink Himalayan salt and pepper.
3. Spread the radishes on a baking sheet in a single layer—roast for 15 minutes, stirring halfway through.
4. Meanwhile, when the radishes have been roasting for about 10 minutes, in a small, light-colored saucepan over medium heat, melt the butter completely, stirring frequently, and season with pink Himalayan salt. Wait for the butter starts to bubble and foam, continue stirring. When the bubbling diminishes a bit, the butter should be a nice nutty brown. The browning process should take about 3 minutes in total.

Transfer the browned butter to a heat-safe container (I use a mug).

5. Remove the radishes from the oven, and divide them between two plates. Spoon the brown butter over the radishes, top with the chopped parsley, and serve.

Nutrition:

Calories: 181

Total Fat: 19g

Carbs: 4g

Protein: 1g

Parmesan and Pork Rind Green Beans

Preparation Time: 5 Minutes

Cooking Time: 15 Minutes

Servings: 2

Ingredients:

- ½ pound fresh green beans
- Two tablespoons crushed pork rinds
- Two tablespoons olive oil
- One tablespoon grated Parmesan cheese
- Pink Himalayan salt
- Freshly ground black pepper

Directions:

1. Preheat the oven to 400°F.

2. In a medium bowl, blend the green beans, pork rinds, olive oil, and Parmesan cheese. Season with pink Himalayan salt and pepper, and toss until the beans are thoroughly coated.

3. Spread the bean mixture on a baking sheet in a single layer and roast for about 15 minutes. At the halfway point, give the pan a little shake to move the beans around, or just stir them.

4. Divide the beans between two plates and serve.

Nutrition:

Calories: 175

Total Fat: 15g

Carbs: 8g Fiber: 3g

Protein: 6g

Pesto Cauliflower Steaks

Preparation Time: 5 Minutes

Cooking Time: 20 Minutes

Servings: 2

Ingredients:

- Two tablespoons olive oil, plus more for brushing
- ½ head cauliflower
- Pink Himalayan salt
- Freshly ground black pepper
- 2 cups fresh basil leaves
- ½ cup grated Parmesan cheese
- ¼ cup almonds
- ½ cup shredded mozzarella cheese

Directions:

1. Preheat the oven to 425°F.

2. Brush a baking sheet by means of olive oil or line with a silicone baking mat.

3. To prep the cauliflower steaks, remove and discard the leaves and

cut the cauliflower into 1-inch-thick slices. You can roast the extra floret crumbles that fall off with the steaks.

4. Place the cauliflower steaks on the arranged baking sheet, and brush them with the olive oil. You want the surface just lightly coated, so it gets caramelized—season with pink Himalayan salt and pepper.

5. Roast the cauliflower steaks for 20 minutes.

6. Meanwhile, put the basil, Parmesan cheese, almonds, and two tablespoons of olive oil in a food processor (or blender) and season with pink Himalayan salt and pepper. Mix until combined.

7. Spread some pesto on top of each cauliflower steak, and top with the mozzarella cheese. Return to the oven and bake until the cheese melts, about 2 minutes.

8. Place the cauliflower steaks on two plates, and serve hot.

Nutrition: Calories: 448

Total Fat: 34gCarbs: 17g

Fiber: 7gProtein: 24g

Tomato, Avocado, and Cucumber Salad

Preparation Time: 5 Minutes

Cooking Time: 0 Minutes

Servings: 2

Ingredients:

- ½ cup grape tomatoes halved

- Four small Persian cucumbers or 1 English cucumber, peeled and finely chopped
- One avocado, finely chopped
- ¼ cup crumbled feta cheese
- Two tablespoons vinaigrette salad dressing
- Pink Himalayan salt
- Freshly ground black pepper

Directions:

1. In a large bowl, blend the tomatoes, cucumbers, avocado, and feta cheese.
2. Add the vinaigrette, and season with pink Himalayan salt and pepper. Toss to combine thoroughly.
3. Divide the salad between two plates and serve.

Nutrition:

Calories: 258

Total Fat: 23g

Carbs: 12g

Protein: 5g

Crunchy Pork Rind Zucchini Sticks

Preparation Time: 5 Minutes

Cooking Time: 25 Minutes

Servings: 2

Ingredients:

- Two medium zucchinis halved lengthwise and seeded
- ¼ cup crushed pork rinds

- ¼ cup grated Parmesan cheese
- Two garlic cloves, minced
- Two tablespoons melted butter
- Pink Himalayan salt
- Freshly ground black pepper
- Olive oil, for drizzling

Directions:

1. Preheat the oven to 400°F.
2. Place the zucchini splits cut-side up on the prepared baking sheet.
3. Toss the pork rinds, Parmesan cheese, garlic, melted butter, and season with pink Himalayan salt and pepper in a bowl. Mix until well combined.
4. Spoon the pork-rind mixture onto each zucchini stick, and drizzle each with a little olive oil.
5. Bake for around 20 minutes, or wait until the topping is golden brown.
6. Switch on the broiler to finish browning the zucchini sticks, 3 to 5 minutes, and serve.

Nutrition:

Calories: 231 Total Fat: 20g

Carbs: 8g Fiber: 2g Protein: 9g

Cauliflower "Potato" Salad

Preparation Time: 10 Minutes

Cooking Time: 25 Minutes

Servings: 2

Ingredients:

- ½ head cauliflower

- One tablespoon olive oil
- Pink Himalayan salt
- Freshly ground black pepper
- 1/3 cup mayonnaise
- One tablespoon mustard
- ¼ cup diced dill pickles
- One teaspoon paprika

Directions:

1. Preheat the oven to 400°F.
2. Cut the cauliflower into 1-inch pieces.
3. Put the cauliflower in a large bowl, then add the olive oil, season with the pink Himalayan salt and pepper, and toss to combine.
4. Spread the cauliflower out on the prepared baking sheet and bake for 25 minutes, or just until the cauliflower begins to brown. Midway through the cooking time, give the pan a couple of shakes or stir so all sides of the cauliflower cook.
5. In a large bowl, blend the cauliflower with the mayonnaise, mustard, and pickles. Sprinkle the paprika on top, and chill in the refrigerator for 3 hours before serving.

Nutrition:

Calories: 386

Total Fat: 37g

Carbs: 13g

Fiber: 5g

Protein: 5g

Loaded Cauliflower Mashed "Potatoes"

Preparation Time: 10 Minutes

Cooking Time: 10 Minutes

Servings: 4

Ingredients:

- One head fresh cauliflower, cut into cubes
- Two garlic cloves, minced
- Six tablespoons butter
- Two tablespoons sour cream
- Pink Himalayan salt
- Freshly ground black pepper
- 1 cup shredded cheese (I use Colby Jack)
- Six bacon slices, cooked and crumbled

Directions:

1. Boil water over high heat.
2. Add the cauliflower. Lessen the heat to medium-low, then simmer for 8 to 10 minutes, until fork-tender.
3. Drain the cauliflower in a colander, and turn it out onto a paper towel-lined plate to soak up the water. Blot to remove any remaining water from the cauliflower pieces. This step is essential; you want to get out as much water as possible so the mash won't be runny.
4. Add the cauliflower into the food processor plus the garlic, butter, sour cream, and season with

pink Himalayan salt and pepper.

5. Mix for about 1 minute, stopping to scrape down the sides of the bowl every 30 seconds.

6. Divide the cauliflower mix evenly among four small serving dishes, and top each with the cheese and bacon crumbles.

7. Serve warm.

Nutrition:

Calories: 757

Total Fat: 38g

Carbs: 17g

Fiber: 6g

Protein: 29g

Pork Rind Nachos

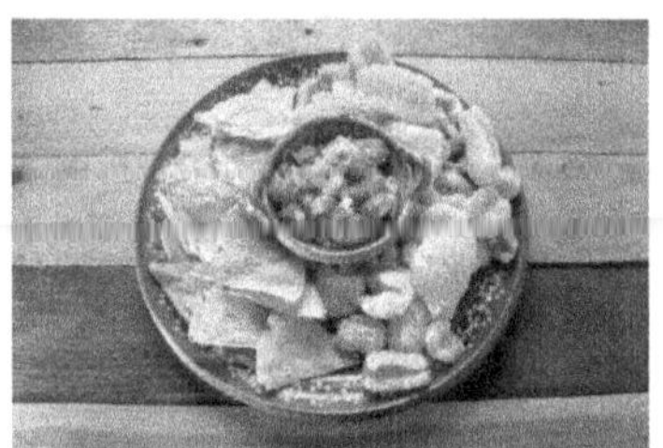

Preparation Time: 10 Minutes

Cooking Time: 10 Minutes

Servings: 4

Ingredients:

- One medium tomato, seeded and chopped
- ¼ white onion, chopped
- One tablespoon chopped fresh cilantro
- One jalapeño pepper, seeded and minced
- One teaspoon minced garlic
- 1½ teaspoons freshly squeezed lime juice
- Sea salt

- Freshly ground black pepper
- 1 (1½-ounce) bag pork rinds
- 2 cups shredded organic Cheddar cheese

Directions:

1. In a small bowl, toss the tomato, onion, garlic, jalapeño, and cilantro.

2. Stir in the lime juice and then season with salt and pepper. Set the salsa aside for at least 1 hour for the flavors to combine. After 1 hour, drain any excess liquid from the salsa.

3. Preheat the oven to 350°F.

4. Arrange the pork rinds in a tight but single layer on the sheet. Sprinkle the cheese over the pork rinds, then top with the salsa.

5. Bake the nachos until the cheese melts and begins to bubble around 15 minutes. Serve hot.

Nutrition:

Calories: 599 Total Fat: 45g

Protein: 41g

Cholesterol: 149mg

Carbohydrates: 6g Fiber: 1g

Sour Cream and Onion Pork Rinds

Preparation Time: 20 Minutes

Cooking Time: 2 Hours and 30 Minutes

Servings: 4

Ingredients:

- 2 pounds of pork skin

- Three tablespoons dried chives
- Three tablespoons sweet cream buttermilk powder
- Two tablespoons onion powder
- One tablespoon garlic powder

Directions:

1. Preheat the oven to 350°F.
2. Using kitchen shears, cut the pork skin into 1-inch squares and place each square skin-side up on the sheet.
3. Bake the skins for 2½ hours.
4. Take it from the oven and set aside until the pork rinds are cool enough to handle.
5. In a large bowl, toss the warm pork rinds with the chives, buttermilk powder, onion powder, and garlic powder. Serve warm or at room temperature.

Nutrition:

Calories: 278

Total Fat: 19g

Protein: 25g

Cholesterol: 90mg

Carbohydrates: 1.5g

Baked Cheddar Chips

Preparation Time: 5 Minutes

Cooking Time: 5 Minutes

Servings: 4

Ingredients:

- 4 cups shredded organic Cheddar cheese
- Sea salt

Directions:

1. Preheat the oven to 350°F.
2. Spread out the cheese lightly on the sheet.
3. Bake for 3 to 5 minutes, regularly checking until the cheese browns but does not burn.
4. Take it away from the oven, then season the cheese with salt.
5. Although the cheese is still warm, use a pizza cutter to cut it into strips or triangles. Let cool before serving.

Nutrition:

Calories: 457

Total Fat: 38g

Protein: 28g

Cholesterol: 119mg

Carbohydrates: 1g

Baked Parmesan Chips

Preparation Time: 5 Minutes

Cooking Time: 5 Minutes

Servings: 4

Ingredients:

- 10 ounces shredded organic Parmesan cheese
- Sea salt

Directions:

1. Preheat the oven to 350°F.
2. Form small Parmesan cheese circles on the sheet.
3. Bake, frequently checking, until the cheese browns but does not burn, 3 to 5 minutes.
4. Take away from the oven and sprinkle the

cheese with the salt. Let cool before serving.

Nutrition:

Calories: 228

Total Fat: 15g

Protein: 23g

Cholesterol: 51mg

Carbohydrates: 2g

Mini Mozzarella Sticks

Preparation Time: 10 Minutes

Cooking Time: 2 Minutes

Servings: 4

Ingredients:

- 1 (1½-ounce) bag pork rinds
- One tablespoon Italian seasoning
- One teaspoon garlic powder
- ¼ teaspoon of sea salt
- ¼ teaspoon freshly ground black pepper
- ¼ cup grated organic Parmesan cheese
- One large free-range egg
- One large free-range egg white
- Ten whole-milk organic mozzarella cheese sticks
- Oil, for frying
- Marinara sauce, for dipping (optional)

Directions:

1. In a food processor, put the pork rinds, Italian seasoning, garlic powder, salt, and pepper. Pulse until you have a breadcrumb-like evenness.

2. Use a spatula for stirring in the Parmesan cheese. Handover some of the

mixtures to a small bowl.

3. In another small bowl, beat together the egg and egg white.

4. Slice each mozzarella stick into two short halves.

5. Dip each mozzarella half into the egg combination, then roll it in the "breading," refilling the breading as needed. Put the coated mozzarella sticks on the baking sheet or plate.

6. Freeze the mozzarella sticks for at least 1 hour.

7. In a large frypan over medium-high heat, heat sufficient oil to cover the bottom of the pan. When the oil is hot, fry the mozzarella sticks for about 1 minute on each side. Serve warm, with a marinara sauce for dipping (if using).

Nutrition:

Calories: 430

Total Fat: 36g

Protein: 29g

Cholesterol: 114mg

Carbohydrates: 2g

Mozzarella Crust Pizza

Preparation Time: 5 Minutes

Cooking Time: 15 Minutes

Servings: 2

Ingredients:

- 2 cups shredded organic mozzarella cheese
- One teaspoon garlic powder
- One teaspoon plus a pinch pizza seasoning, divided

- ½ cup tomato sauce
- Grated organic Parmesan cheese

Directions:

1. Preheat the oven to 400°F.
2. Place the mozzarella on the sheet in an even layer to form a large rectangle with no holes.
3. Sprinkle the garlic powder and a pinch of pizza seasoning over the cheese. Bake and wait until the cheese is melted and browned all around the edges, 12 to 15 minutes.
4. Take it from the oven and set aside to cool for 3 minutes.
5. Spread the tomato sauce over the top of the crust, and then sprinkle it with the Parmesan cheese and the remaining one teaspoon of pizza seasoning. Coming back the pizza to the oven for about 1 minute. Slice and serve hot.

Nutrition:

Calories: 324 Total Fat: 20g

Protein: 33g Cholesterol: 60mg

Carbohydrates: 4g

Mini Salami and Cheese Pizzas

Preparation Time: 5 Minutes

Cooking Time: 1 Minute

Servings: 1

Ingredients:

- 4 slices Genoa salami

- Four tablespoons Rhode Island Red Marinara Sauce, divided
- Four tablespoons shredded organic mozzarella cheese, divided
- Pizza seasoning

Directions:

1. Preheat the oven to broil.
2. Layout the salami slices on the sheet put space between each one. Top each with one tablespoon of marinara. Then sprinkle one tablespoon of mozzarella on each pizza and add a pinch of pizza seasoning.
3. Place the pizzas under the broiler until the cheese bubbles, about 1 minute. Serve.

Nutrition:

Calories: 259

Total Fat: 19g

Saturated Fat: 8g

Protein: 17g

Cholesterol: 53mg

Carbohydrates: 4g

Chicken Ramen Dip

Preparation Time: 5 Minutes

Cooking Time: 0 Minutes

Servings: 6

Ingredients:

- 6 ounces organic sour cream
- ¼ cup organic cream cheese, at room temperature
- Two tablespoons mayonnaise

- One seasoning packet from a package of chicken ramen or spicy ramen

Directions:

1. In a medium bowl, place the sour cream, cream cheese, mayonnaise, and seasoning.
2. With a hand mixer or immersion blender, blend everything until well combined.
3. Cover the bowl and refrigerate the dip for at least 1 hour, or overnight, for the flavors to meld.

Nutrition:

Calories: 156

Total Fat: 16g

Protein: 3g

Cholesterol: 36mg

Carbohydrates: 1g

Creamy Crab Dip

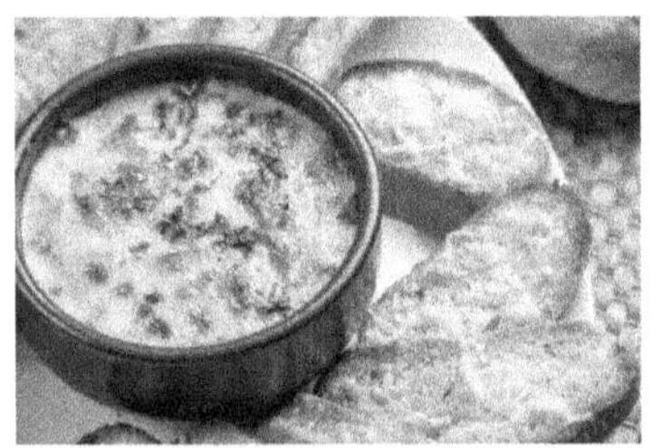

Preparation Time: 10 Minutes

Cooking Time: 30 Minutes

Servings: 6

Ingredients:

- Grass-fed butter, at room temperature
- 1-pound lump crabmeat
- ½ cup diced red bell pepper
- 1 cup organic cream cheese
- One tablespoon mayonnaise

- One tablespoon horseradish
- Two teaspoons Cajun seasoning
- 1/8 teaspoon garlic salt

Directions:

1. Preheat the oven to 350°F.
2. Grease a small baking dish with butter.
3. In a medium bowl, blend the crabmeat, red bell pepper, cream cheese, mayonnaise, horseradish, Cajun seasoning, and garlic salt until well blended.
4. Transfer the dip to the baking dish, then bake it for 30 minutes. Serve warm.

Nutrition:

Calories: 292

Total Fat: 31g

Protein: 21g

Cholesterol: 129mg

Carbohydrates: 2g

Bacon-Whiskey Caramelized Onion Dip

Preparation Time: 10 Minutes

Cooking Time: 25 Minutes

Servings: 6

Ingredients:

- Two tablespoons bacon fat
- Two onions halved lengthwise and cut crosswise into ¼-inch-thick slices
- Three teaspoons whiskey, divided
- Three tablespoons water, divided
- 1 cup organic sour cream

- ½ cup organic cream cheese, at room temperature
- ½ teaspoon of sea salt
- ¼ teaspoon garlic powder

Directions:

1. In a frypan, dissolve the bacon fat over medium-low heat.

2. Put the onions in the hot fat and cook for 3 minutes.

3. With a wooden spoon to break apart any onion pieces, still sticking together and continue cooking the onions, stirring every few minutes, for 20 minutes.

4. When the onions begin to get a little dry and stick to the skillet, stir in 1 teaspoon of whiskey. Alternate adding one teaspoon of whiskey and one tablespoon of water until you've used all the whiskey, then use water as needed.

5. When the onions are soft, sweet, and very brown, transfer them to a bowl and refrigerate until cold.

6. In a blender, combine the sour cream, cream cheese, salt, and garlic powder. Blend until smooth and well mixed.

7. Add the cold onions to the blender, and pulse to achieve your desired consistency. Handover the dip to an airtight container and refrigerate for at least 1 hour. Stir the dip just before serving.

Nutrition:

Calories: 362

Total Fat: 36g

Protein: 4g

Cholesterol: 70mg

Carbohydrates: 4g

Creamy Dill Deviled Eggs

Preparation Time: 10 Minutes

Cooking Time: 30 Minutes

Servings: 6

Ingredients:

- 12 large free-range eggs
- Six tablespoons mayonnaise
- One tablespoon dried dill
- One teaspoon sea salt

Directions:

1. Place each whole egg in the cup of a mini-muffin tin.

2. Turn the oven to 325°F and place the muffin tin in the oven (do not preheat the oven). Bake the eggs for 30 minutes.

3. Prepare a large bowl of ice water. Put the eggs in the ice water and shake from side to side, they slightly crack each other. Once they are cool, peel the eggs, and cut each one in half lengthwise. Scoop the yolks into a small bowl.

4. Add the mayonnaise, dill, and salt to the bowl with the yolks and mix until smooth.

5. Place the yolk mixture in a small zipper-top plastic bag. Slice one

corner of the bag at the bottom and pipe the filling into the egg halves. Serve

Nutrition:

Calories: 202

Total Fat: 15g

Protein: 14g

Cholesterol: 376mg

Carbohydrates: 3g

Roasted Pesto Pepper Poppers

Preparation Time: 10 Minutes

Cooking Time: 20 Minutes

Servings: 6

Ingredients:

- 12 mini bell peppers, halved lengthwise and seeded
- ½ cup prepared pesto
- ¼ cup organic goat cheese
- ¼ cup organic cream cheese, at room temperature
- Two tablespoons diced shallot
- One teaspoon cayenne pepper sauce
- One tablespoon fresh thyme leaf

Directions:

1. Preheat the oven to 350°F.
2. Line a rimmed baking sheet with parchment paper.
3. Lay the mini pepper halves, cut-side up, on the sheet.
4. In a small bowl, mix the pesto, goat cheese, cream cheese, shallot, and cayenne pepper sauce.

5. Fill the pepper halves with the pesto and cheese mixture. Sprinkle them with the thyme.

6. Bake for 20 minutes. Serve hot.

Nutrition:

Calories: 172

Total Fat: 15g

Protein: 4g

Cholesterol: 18mg

Carbohydrates: 5g

Macadamia Shortbread Cookies

Preparation Time: 5 Minutes

Cooking Time: 30 Minutes

Servings: 16

Ingredients:

- 2 cups almond flour

- ¾ cup macadamia nuts, chopped

- 3 oz. dark chocolate, chopped

- ½ cup butter softened

- 2/3 cup erythritol

- ½ tsp. vanilla extract

- ½ tsp. salt

- 1 tbsp. coconut oil

Directions:

1. Preheat the oven to 300 F. Make a cookie sheet and line with a silicone mat.

2. Beat butter and erythritol in a bowl until fluffy. Add salt and vanilla.

3. Add almond flour and macadamia nuts and beat until combined. Transfer to the sheet and roll out until about ¼ inch thick. Cut the

cookies with the pizza cutter.

4. Bake for 30 minutes. Let cool and serve

Nutrition:

Calories 207

Fat 19.7 g

Carbs 6 g

Protein 3.8 g

Chocolate Muffins

Preparation Time: 5 Minutes

Cooking Time: 30 Minutes

Servings: 16

Ingredients:

- Three eggs
- 1 cup cacao powder
- ½ cup coconut flour
- 4½ oz. cacao butter, melted
- 2 cups pumpkin, cooked, chopped
- ½ cup of coconut oil
- ½ cup collagen protein powder
- 3 tsp. vanilla extract
- 2 tsp. apple cider vinegar
- 1 tsp. baking soda
- 4 tbsp. erythritol
- Pinch of salt

Directions:

1. Preheat the oven to 350 F.
2. Add eggs, cacao powder, coconut flour, cacao butter, pumpkin, coconut oil, vanilla, vinegar, soda, sweetener, and salt to a blender and blitz until smooth.
3. Add collagen and process again until combined.
4. Transfer the batter to a muffin pan and spread

evenly—Cook for about 30 minutes. Let cool and serve.

Nutrition:

Calories 111

Fat 9.9 g

Carbs 4 g

Protein 2.8 g

No-Bake Coconut Cookies

Preparation Time: 5 Minutes

Cooking Time: 5 Minutes

Servings: 8

Ingredients:

- 2 tsp. vanilla
- 3 cups coconut, shredded
- ½ cup xylitol or any keto-friendly sweetener
- 3/8 cup coconut oil

- salt to taste
- shredded coconut, melted chocolate, cocoa/carob powder, or crushed nuts for toppings

Directions:

1. Add all fixings to a blender and process until the mixture is nicely blended.
2. When done, transfer the mixture from the blender and prepare cookies in any shape.
3. Decorate each cookie with crushed nuts, cocoa/carob powder, shredded coconut, melted chocolate, or just leave them plain.
4. Set cookies on a plate and allow them to firm up at room temperature.

5. Cool in the fridge or serve at room temperature.

Nutrition:

Calories 328

Fat 29.6 g

Carbs 4.1 g

Protein 2.1 g

Coconut Blondies

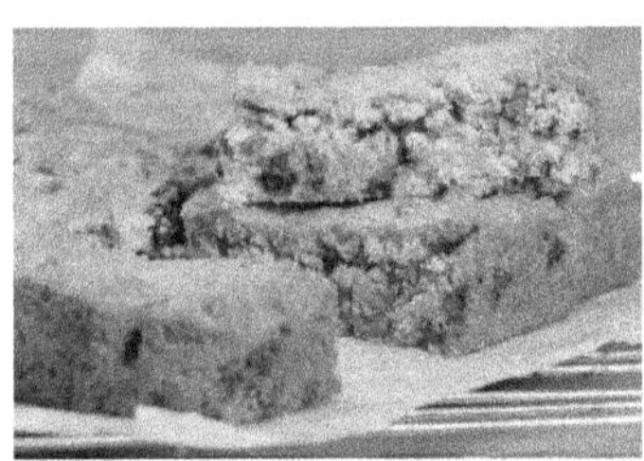

Preparation Time: 5 Minutes

Cooking Time: 30 Minutes

Servings: 9

Ingredients:

- ¼ cup of coconut milk
- ¼ tsp. baking powder
- ½ cup erythritol, or sugar substitute
- Four eggs
- 1 tbsp. vanilla extract
- ½ cup coconut, desiccated
- ½ cup unsalted butter softened
- ½ cup coconut flour
- ¼ tsp. salt

Directions:

1. Preheat the oven to 350 F.
2. Combine butter and erythritol and mix well until even.
3. Add eggs at a time, blending into the batter bit by bit.
4. Add coconut milk and vanilla extract, then beat thoroughly until the desired smoothness is achieved.

5. Add coconut flour to the mixture and desiccated coconut, salt, and baking powder, then stir gently until smooth. The mixture should not be too thick; if it is, add a little more coconut milk.

6. When done, spoon the batter into the prepared baking pan and allow it to bake until golden and firm, about 25-30 minutes.

7. When baked through, cool in the baking tin for 30 minutes, then cut and serve.

Nutrition:

Calories 189

Fat 17 g

Carbs 6 g

Protein 4 g

Chocolate and Hazelnut Spread

Preparation Time: 5 Minutes

Cooking Time: 5 Minutes

Servings: 6

Ingredients:

- 1 tsp. vanilla extract
- ¼ cup of coconut oil
- 5 oz. hazelnuts
- 2 tbsp. cocoa powder
- 1 tsp. erythritol
- 1 oz. butter, unsalted

Directions:

1. Put hazelnuts in a hot, dry pan and roast until golden.
2. When roasted through, shed hazelnuts shells by putting them in a kitchen towel and rubbing them gently.
3. When done, put hazelnuts in a blender along with all remaining ingredients and process until smooth.

Nutrition:

Calories 271

Fat 28 g

Carbs 2 g

Protein 4 g

Cinnamon and Cardamom Fat Bombs

Preparation Time: 5 Minutes

Cooking Time: 35 Minutes

Servings: 10

Ingredients:

- ¼ tsp. ground green cardamom
- 3 oz. butter, unsalted
- ½ tsp. vanilla extract
- ¼ tsp. ground cinnamon

- ½ cup coconut, unsweetened, shredded

Directions:

1. Warm butter to room temperature and roast shredded coconut in a pan over medium heat until slightly browned. Let it cool for a while.
2. Add spices to a bowl with butter and half of the shredded coconut, refrigerate until slightly firm for at least 5-10 minutes.
3. When done, form into walnut-size balls and roll them in the other half of the shredded coconut.
4. When ready, put balls in the freezer or refrigerator.

Nutrition:

Calories 90

Fat 10 g

Carbs 0.4 g

Protein 0.4 g

Coconut Panna Cotta with Cream & Caramel

Preparation Time: 5 Minutes

Cooking Time: 1 Hour and 10 Minutes

Servings: 4

Ingredients:

- Four eggs
- 1/3 cup erythritol, for caramel
- 2 cups of coconut milk
- 1 tbsp. vanilla extract
- 1 tbsp. lemon zest
- ½ cup erythritol, for custard
- 2 cups heavy whipping cream
- Mint leaves, to serve

Directions:

1. In a deep pan, heat the erythritol for the caramel. Add two tbsp. of water and bring to a boil. Lower the heat and cook until the caramel turns to a golden-brown color.

2. Divide among four metal tins, set aside, and let it cool. In a bowl, mix the eggs, remaining erythritol, lemon zest, and vanilla. Beat in the coconut milk until combined.

3. Pour the custard into each caramel-lined ramekin and put them into a deep baking tin. Fill over the way with the remaining hot water—Bake at 350 F. for around 45 minutes.

4. Take out the ramekins with tongs and refrigerate them for at least 3 hours. Run a knife slowly around the edges to invert onto a dish. Serve with dollops of whipped cream and scattered with mint leaves.

Nutrition:

Calories 268 Fat 31 g

Carbs 2.5 g Protein 6.5 g

Blueberry Ice Balls

Preparation Time: 5 Minutes

Cooking Time: 12 Minutes

Servings: 4

Ingredients:

- ½ tsp. vanilla extract
- Two packets gelatin, without sugar

- 2 tbsp. heavy whipping cream
- 2 cups of water
- 3 tbsp. mashed blueberries
- 2 cups crushed ice
- 1 cup of cold water

Directions:

1. Boil the water over medium heat and dissolve the gelatin inside. Transfer to a blender and add the remaining ingredients. Pulse until smooth and make balls.
2. Freeze them for 3 hours.

Nutrition:

Calories 142

Fat 9 g

Carbs 7.8 g

Protein 3.5 g

Raspberry Coconut Cheesecake

Preparation Time: 5 Minutes

Cooking Time: 50 Minutes

Servings: 1

Ingredients:

Crust:

- ¼ cup xylitol
- 3 cups desiccated coconut
- Two egg whites
- 1 tsp. coconut oil
- ¼ cup butter, melted

Filling:

- 6 oz. raspberries
- 3 tbsp. lemon juice
- 2 cups xylitol
- 1 cup whipped cream
- Zest of 1 lemon
- 3 cups cream cheese

Directions:

1. Grease the pan with oil and line with parchment paper.
2. In a bowl, mix all crust ingredients and pour the crust into the pan. Preheat the oven to 330 F. Bake for 30 minutes, then let cool.
3. Meanwhile, beat the cream cheese with an electric mixer until soft. Add the lemon juice, zest, and xylitol. Put the whipped cream into the cheese cream mixture.
4. Gently fold in the raspberries and spoon the filling into the baked and cooled crust. Chill for 4 hours.

Nutrition:

Calories 376

Fat 32 g

Carbs 6 g

Protein 7 g

Avocado & Berry Fruit Dessert

Preparation Time: 5 Minutes

Cooking Time: 5 Minutes

Servings: 4

Ingredients:

- ½ cup walnuts, toasted
- One avocado, chopped
- 1 cup cream cheese, softened
- 1 cup fresh blueberries
- 1 cup fresh raspberries
- 1 cup fresh blackberries

Directions:

1. Divide half of the cream cheese, half of the mixed berries, half of the walnuts, and half of the avocado among

four dessert glasses. Repeat the layering process for a second time to finish the ingredients.

2. Cover the glasses with plastic wrap and refrigerate for 1 hour until quite firm.

Nutrition:

Calories 322

Fat 28.3 g

Carbs 6.5 g

Protein 9 g

Moist Avocado Brownies

Preparation Time: 10 Minutes

Cooking Time: 35 Minutes

Servings: 9

Ingredients:

- Two avocados, mashed
- Two eggs
- 1 tsp. baking powder
- 2 tbsp. swerve
- 1/3 cup chocolate chips, melted
- 4 tbsp. coconut oil, melted
- 2/3 cup unsweetened cocoa powder

Directions:

1. Preheat the oven to 325 F.
2. In a mixing bowl, mix all dry ingredients.
3. In another bowl, mix avocado and eggs until well combined.
4. Slowly add dry mixture to the wet along with melted chocolate and coconut oil. Mix well.
5. Pour batter into a greased baking pan and bake for 30-35 minutes.
6. Slice and serve.

Nutrition:

Calories 207

Fat 18 g

Carbs 11 g

Protein 3.8 g

Choco Peanut Cookies

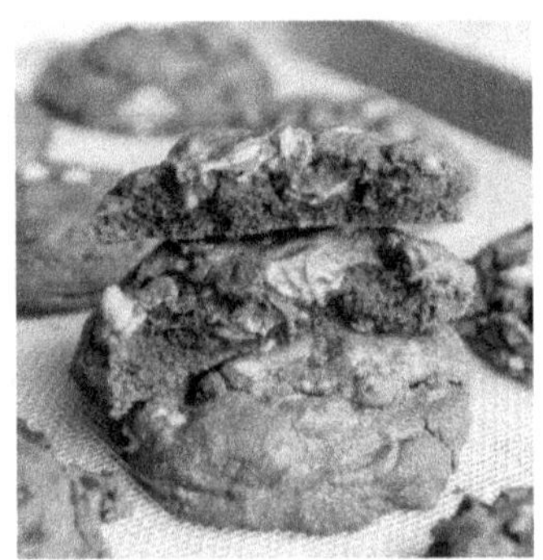

Preparation Time: 10 Minutes

Cooking Time: 10 Minutes

Servings: 24

Ingredients:

- 1 cup peanut butter
- 1 tsp. baking soda
- 2 tsp. vanilla
- 1 tbsp. butter, melted

- Two eggs
- 2 tbsp. unsweetened cocoa powder
- 2/3 cup erythritol
- 1 1/3 cups almond flour

Directions:

1. Preheat the oven to 350 F.
2. Add all fixings to the mixing bowl and stir to combine.
3. Make 2-inch balls from the mixture, put on the greased baking tray, and gently press each ball down with a fork.
4. Bake in the oven for 8-10 minutes.
5. Serve and enjoy.

Nutrition:

Calories 110 Fat 9 g

Carbs 9 g Protein 4.6 g

Maple and Pecan Bars

Preparation Time: 10 Minutes

Cooking Time: 25 Minutes

Servings: 12

Ingredients:

- ½ cup flaxseed meal
- 2 cups pecans, toasted and crushed
- 1 cup almond flour
- ½ cup of coconut oil
- ¼ tsp. stevia
- ½ cup coconut, shredded
- ¼ cup "maple syrup" (see below)

For the maple syrup:

- ¼ cup erythritol
- 2¼ tsp. coconut oil
- 1 tbsp. butter
- ¼ tsp. xanthan gum
- ¾ cup of water
- 2 tsp. maple extract
- ½ tsp. vanilla extract

Directions:

1. In a heatproof bowl, mix the butter with 2¼ tsp. coconut oil and xanthan gum, stir, put in a microwave, and heat for 1 minute.
2. Add the erythritol, water, maple, and vanilla extract, stir well, and heat in the microwave for 1 minute. In a bowl, mix the flaxseed meal with coconut and almond flour, and stir.
3. Add the pecans and stir again.
4. Add the ¼ cup "maple syrup," stevia, and ½ cup coconut oil and stir well. Spread this in a baking dish, press fine, put into an oven at 350°

F., and bake for 25 minutes.

5. Set aside to cool down, cut into 12 bars, and serve.

Nutrition:

Calories 300

Fat 30 g

Carbs 2 g

Protein 5 g

CHAPTER 7:

Lunch

Lime Chicken with Savoy Cabbage

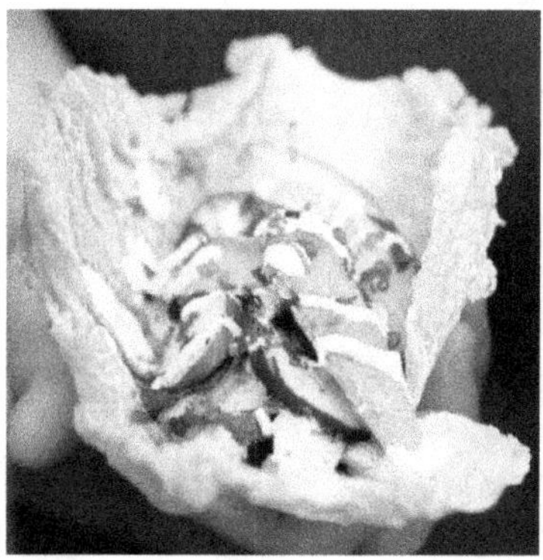

Preparation Time: 10 Minutes

Cooking Time: 7 Hours

Servings: 4

Ingredients:

- Eight chicken thighs, skinless
- 2 cups Savoy cabbage, chopped
- One stalk celery, diced
- One medium onion, diced
- 1 tbsp ginger, grated
- ½ cup chicken stock
- Two limes
- 1 tsp salt
- 1 tsp black pepper
- Extra virgin olive oil
- Spicy squash noodles for serving

Directions:

1. Place 4 tbsp extra virgin olive oil in a slow cooker, spread around the bottom. Add the ginger and onions.
2. Slice lime into ½" thick circles. Place chicken in the bottom of a slow

cooker, and sprinkle with ½ tsp salt and ½ tsp black pepper. Top with lime slices

3. On top of those, place the celery and cabbage.

4. Pour in chicken stock, then cook on Low for 7 hours.

5. Serve with Spicy Squash Noodles.

Nutrition:

Calories 273

Carbs 5.7 g

Fat 12 g

Protein 34 g

Middle Eastern Lamb Zucchini Casserole

Preparation Time: 20 Minutes

Cooking Time: 7 Hours

Servings: 6

Ingredients:

- Four zucchinis, peeled
- 1 lb. ground lamb
- ½ cup coconut cream
- Two eggs
- ¼ cup Parmesan
- ½ tsp cinnamon
- ½ tsp cloves
- ½ tsp cumin
- 1 tsp salt
- 1 tsp black pepper
- Extra virgin olive oil

Directions:

1. Use a mandolin, thinly-slice zucchini lengthwise.

2. Heat 3 tbsp extra virgin olive oil in the skillet. Add lamb, cinnamon, cloves, and cumin. Brown.

3. Combine coconut cream with egg, salt, and black pepper—coat

slow cooker with olive oil, place ¼ of zucchini strips on the slow cooker's bottom.

4. Next, brush coconut cream mixture on zucchini.

5. Place another layer of zucchini and half the remaining coconut cream, top with lamb, another layer of zucchini, remaining coconut cream.

6. Cook on Low for 7 hours.

Nutrition:

Calories 203

Carbs 4.7 g

Fat 10 g

Protein 25 g

Ginger Steak Broccoli

Preparation Time: 10 Minutes

Cooking Time: 4 Hours

Servings: 4

Ingredients:

- 1 lb. sirloin steak
- 3 cups broccoli florets (frozen okay)
- 1 cup low-sodium beef stock
- 1 tbsp grated ginger
- ½ tsp thyme
- 1 tsp salt
- 1 tsp black pepper
- Extra virgin olive oil

Directions:

- Slice sirloin steak against the grain into ½" wide strips.
- Place 4 tbsp extra virgin olive oil in a skillet, add steak, and brown for a minute on each side.

- Place steak, broccoli florets, along with ginger, beef stock, and soy sauce in a slow cooker.
- Cook on medium-high for 4 hours.
- Enjoy alone or with cauliflower rice.

Nutrition:

Calories 273 Carbs 6 g

Fat 11 g Protein 37 g

Sodium 714 mg

BLT Chicken Salad

Preparation Time: 20 Minutes

Cooking Time: 4 Hours

Servings: 4

Ingredients:

- 4 x 4oz chicken breast
- 2 cup low-sodium chicken broth
- Eight slices bacon
- 2 cups romaine lettuce
- One tomato, diced
- 1 tsp salt
- 1 tsp black pepper
- ¼ cup organic mayonnaise
- Extra virgin olive oil

Directions:

1. Coat slow cooker with a little olive oil, and set on high.
2. Tenderize chicken breast, and sprinkle each chicken breast with salt and black pepper.
3. Wrap each chicken breast with bacon, and place it in a slow cooker.
4. Cook chicken breast on high for 4 hours.
5. Place mayonnaise with 1 tsp black pepper and 4 tbsp extra virgin olive

oil in a blender. Mix until smooth.

6. Combine lettuce, tomato in a bowl, and toss with mayo dressing.

7. Top salad with chicken breast and serve.

Nutrition:

Calories 366 Carbs 6 g

Fat 19 g Protein 43 g

Sodium 1183 mg

Figs and Goat Cheese-Stuffed Chicken

Preparation Time: 20 Minutes

Cooking Time: 8 Hours

Servings: 4

Ingredients:

- 4 x 4oz chicken breasts

- 4 figs

- ½ cup goat cheese, crumbled

- 1 tsp salt

- 1 tsp black pepper

- Extra virgin olive oil

Directions:

1. Combine 3 tbsp olive oil, salt, black pepper in a bowl, and rub onto chicken breasts. Marinate for an hour.

2. Remove fig skin, and slice figs into ½" pieces. Combine with goat cheese.

3. Turn slow cooker to Low.

4. Place plastic wrap over chicken breasts and pound with a mallet until each breast is approximately ¼" thick (or ask your butcher to do it).

5. Scoop a quarter of the cheese-fig mixture into the chicken, roll up chicken breast, and place in a slow cooker.

6. Repeat for each chicken breast.

7. Cook on low for 8 hours.

8. Serve with a green salad.

Nutrition:

Calories 369 Carbs 7 g

Fat 18 g Protein 46 g

Sodium 811 mg

Carne Asada

Preparation Time: 10 Minutes

Cooking Time: 8 Hours

Servings: 8

Ingredients:

- 4 lb. chuck roast
- 1 onion, chopped
- Four limes, juiced
- ½ cup cilantro, minced
- Eight cloves garlic, minced
- 2 tsp paprika
- 2 tsp oregano
- 2 tsp cumin
- 2 tsp salt
- 1 tsp black pepper

Directions:

1. Rinse pot roast and pat dry.

2. Combine remaining fixings in a blender, and mix until well combined.

3. Brush slow cooker with extra virgin olive oil, and set on high.

4. Coat pot roast with cilantro topping.

5. Place in a slow cooker, and cook for 8 hours.

6. Serve with Cauliflower Rice.

Nutrition:

Calories 506

Carbs 3 g

Fat 19 g

Protein 75 g

Sodium 733 mg

Amazing Pulled Pork

Preparation Time: 25 Minutes

Cooking Time: 8 Hours

Servings: 8

Ingredients:

- 5 lb. pork shoulder
- 2 tbsp mustard
- 2 cups tomato purée
- 6 Medjool Dates, pitted
- ½ tsp cloves, ground
- ½ tsp cinnamon
- 2 tsp salt
- Extra virgin olive oil
- Tortilla Wraps
- Eight eggs
- 1 tbsp coconut flour
- ½ tsp salt

Directions:

1. Place pitted dates in a blender, mix until paste forms, add tomato purée, cinnamon, salt, black pepper, and mix. Combine mustard, blended tomato puree, cloves, cinnamon, salt, and mix.

2. Place pork shoulder in a slow cooker, pour the sauce into a slow cooker, and coat pork shoulder—Cook pork for 8 hours on high.

3. Once the pork is cooked, use a fork to shred.

4. For tortilla wraps, whisk eggs, add milk and

flour, and mix until well combined.

5. Heat 4 tbsp oil in a skillet on medium-high.

6. Pour 1/8th of the mixture into skillet and cook each side 30 seconds.

7. Spoon pork mixture into egg tortilla and serve.

Nutrition:

Calories 777 Carbs 8 g

Fat 55 g Protein 59 g

Sodium 835 mg

Braised Pork Belly

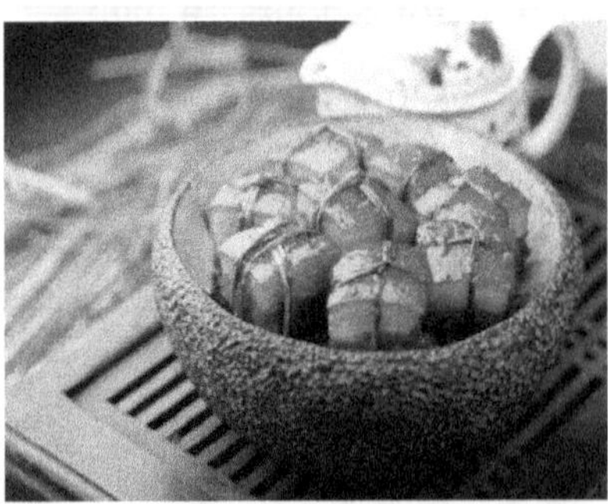

Preparation Time: 10 Minutes

Cooking Time: 4 Hours

Servings: 8

Ingredients:

- 1 lb. pork belly
- Two medium onions, diced
- 1 tsp Dijon mustard
- ½ cup apple sauce
- 1 tsp black pepper
- 1 tsp salt

Directions:

1. Heat extra virgin olive oil in the skillet, add onion, sauté for a minute.

2. Place onion in a slow cooker, add pork belly, apple sauce—cook on high for 4 hours.

3. Serve with Walnut Cabbage Salad.

Nutrition:

Calories 278

Carbs 3.5 g

Fat 15 g

Protein 26 g

Sodium 1214 mg

Peppercorn Short Ribs

Preparation Time: 10 Minutes

Cooking Time: 4 Hours

Servings: 8

Ingredients:

- 4 lbs. short ribs, bone-in
- Eight peppercorns
- 2 cups low-sodium beef
- One onion, diced
- Two carrots, peeled, diced
- Two celery stalks, diced
- Four cloves, minced
- 1 tsp thyme
- 1 tsp rosemary
- Two bay leaves
- 2 tsp salt
- 2 tsp black pepper
- Extra virgin olive oil

Directions:

1. Heat extra virgin olive oil in a skillet. Add onions and garlic, and sauté until brown.
2. Place onion mixture in a slow cooker, add short ribs, carrots, celery stalk, cloves, thyme, rosemary, peppercorns, bay leaves, salt, and black pepper.
3. Cook on high for 4 hours.

Nutrition:

Calories 520 Carbs 3.7 g

Fat 24 g Protein 67 g

Sodium 923 mg

Spicy Italian Sausage and Zucchini Noodles

Preparation Time: 20 Minutes

Cooking Time: 4 Hours

Servings: 6

Ingredients:

- 6 Spicy Italian pork sausages
- One onion, peeled and diced
- 2 cups low-sodium chicken stock
- One tomato, diced
- Four zucchinis, peeled
- 1 tsp oregano
- 1 tsp salt
- 1 tsp black pepper
- Extra virgin olive oil

Directions:

1. Coat slow cooker with a little extra virgin olive oil, and set to high.
2. Slice sausage into ½" thick rounds, and place in a slow cooker.
3. Heat 3 tbsp extra virgin olive oil in a skillet, add onion and garlic, sauté for a minute, and add to slow cooker.
4. Add tomatoes, oregano, and a tsp of salt and black pepper along with the chicken stock, cover, and cook for 4 hours.
5. Using Mandolin, slice zucchini vertically to create thin Zucchini Noodles.
6. Top zucchini noodles with Spicy Italian Sausage and serve.

Nutrition:

Calories 254 Carbs 8.5 g

Fat 14 g Protein 24 g

Sodium 1044 mg

Meaty Cauliflower Lasagna

Preparation Time: 20 Minutes

Cooking Time: 5 Hours

Servings: 8

Ingredients:

- 1 lb. ground beef
- One small cauliflower head
- One red onion, diced
- Four cloves garlic, minced
- 2 cups crushed tomato
- 1 cup Mozzarella, shredded
- One egg
- 1 tsp oregano
- One bay leaf
- 1 tsp black pepper
- 1 tsp salt
- Extra virgin olive oil

Directions:

1. Brush slow cooker with olive oil, and set the slow cooker on medium-high.
2. Separate cauliflower into florets, peel the outer layer of cauliflower stem and dice stem.
3. Place cauliflower in the food processor, pulse into rice-like granules, crack an egg into cauliflower, and mix along with ½ tsp of salt.
4. Place 3 tbsp olive oil in a skillet, add ground beef, brown, add crushed tomatoes, oregano, bay leaf, black pepper, and ½ tsp salt, mix.
5. Place ½ cauliflower mixture in a slow cooker, next layer 1/3

of the beef mixture and ½ of cheese, place remaining cauliflower on top

6. Spoon remaining sauce on top of the cauliflower, sprinkle with remaining cheese.

7. Cook on medium-high for 5 hours.

Nutrition:

Calories 342 Carbs 8.2 g

Fat 14 g Protein 45 g

Sodium 681 mg

Chili Verde

Preparation Time: 10 Minutes

Cooking Time: 7 Hours

Servings: 8

Ingredients:

- 1½ lbs. pork shoulder
- ½ lb. sirloin, cubed
- 4 Anaheim chiles, stemmed
- Six cloves garlic, minced
- ½ cup cilantro, chopped
- Two onions, peeled and sliced
- Two tomatoes, chopped.
- 1 tbsp tomato paste
- One lime
- 1 tbsp cumin
- 1 tbsp oregano
- Extra virgin olive oil

Directions:

1. Slice pork shoulder into ½" cubes, and set slow cooker to medium. Heat oil in a frying pan, add onions, Anaheim chilies, garlic, and sauté for 2 minutes.

2. Place skillet mixture into a slow cooker, add pork shoulder, sirloin, and stir.

3. Add tomatoes, cilantro, tomato paste, cumin, oregano, and salt to the pot.

4. Cover and cook for 7 hours.

5. Squeeze a little lime in each bowl when serving.

Nutrition:

Calories 262

Carbs 6 g

Fat 16 g

Protein 23 g

Sodium 63 mg

Pork & Bacon Parcels

Preparation Time: 5 Minutes

Cooking Time: 40 Minutes

Servings: 4

Ingredients:

- Four bacon strips
- 2 tbsp fresh parsley, chopped
- Four pork loin chops, boneless
- 1/3 cup cottage cheese
- 1 tbsp olive oil
- One onion, chopped
- 1 tbsp garlic powder
- Two tomatoes, chopped
- 1/3 cup chicken stock
- Salt and black pepper, to taste

Directions:

1. Arrange a bacon strip on top of each pork chop, divide the parsley,

and cottage cheese on top.

2. Roll each pork piece and secure it with toothpicks.

3. Set a pan over medium heat and warm oil, cook the pork parcels until browned, and remove to a plate.

4. Add in the onion, and cook for 5 minutes.

5. Pour in the chicken stock and garlic powder, and cook for 3 minutes.

6. Get rid of the toothpicks from the rolls and return them to the pan.

7. Stir in black pepper, salt, parsley, and tomatoes, bring to a boil, set heat to medium-low, and cook for 25 minutes while covered. Serve.

Nutrition:

Cal 433;

Net Carbs 6.8g;

Fat 23g;

Protein 44.6g

Yummy Spareribs in Béarnaise Sauce

Preparation Time: 5 Minutes

Cooking Time: 30 Minutes

Servings: 4

Ingredients:

- 3 tbsp butter, melted
- Four egg yolks, beaten
- 2 tbsp chopped tarragon
- 2 tsp white wine vinegar
- ½ tsp onion powder
- Salt and black pepper to taste
- 4 tbsp butter

- 2 lb. spareribs, divided into 16

Directions:

1. In a bowl, whisk butter gradually into the egg yolks until evenly mixed.
2. In another bowl, combine tarragon, white wine vinegar, and onion powder.
3. Mix into the egg mixture and season with salt and black pepper; set aside.
4. Melt the butter in a skillet over medium heat. Season the spareribs on both sides with salt and pepper.
5. Cook in the butter on both sides until brown with a crust, minutes.
6. Divide the spareribs between plates and serve with béarnaise sauce to the side and some braised asparagus.

Nutrition:

Cal 878;

Net Carbs 1g;

Fat 78g;

Protein 41g

Salisbury Steak

Preparation Time: 5 Minutes

Cooking Time: 25 Minutes

Servings: 6

Ingredients:

- 2 pounds ground beef
- 1 tbsp onion flakes
- ¾ almond flour
- ¼ cup beef broth
- 1 tbsp chopped parsley
- 1 tbsp Worcestershire sauce

Directions:

1. Combine all ingredients in a bowl.
2. Mix well and make six patties out of the mixture.
3. Arrange on a lined baking sheet.
4. Bake at 375 F for about minutes. Serve.

Nutrition:

Cal 354;

Net Carbs 2.5g;

Fat 28g;

Protein 27g

Delicious Pork Stew

Preparation Time: 5 Minutes

Cooking Time: 1 Hour and 20 Minutes

Servings: 12

Ingredients:

- Two tablespoons coconut oil
- 4 pounds pork, cubed
- Salt and black pepper to the taste
- Two tablespoons ghee
- Three garlic cloves, minced
- ¾ cup beef stock
- ¾ cup apple cider vinegar
- Three carrots, chopped
- One cabbage head, shredded
- ½ cup green onion, chopped
- 1 cup whipping cream

Directions:

1. Heat a pan with the ghee and the oil over medium-high heat, add pork and brown it for a

few minutes on each side.

2. Add vinegar and stock, stir well and bring to a simmer.

3. Add cabbage, garlic, salt and pepper, stir, cover, and cook for 1 hour.

4. Add carrots and green onions, stir and cook for 15 minutes more.

5. Add whipping cream, stir for 1 minute, divide between plates and serve.

6. **Enjoy!**

Nutrition:

Calories 400

Fat 25

Fiber 3

Carbs 6

Protein 43

Asian Ground Pork Bowl with Fried Eggs

Preparation Time: 5 Minutes

Cooking Time: 20 Minutes

Servings: 6

Ingredients:

- Three tablespoons sesame oil
- Six eggs
- 1 ½ pounds ground pork
- 1/2-pound ground chicken
- One teaspoon ginger-garlic paste
- One teaspoon ground coriander
- 1/2 Chinese cabbage, shredded
- One red onion, chopped
- Four tablespoons rice wine

- One teaspoon hot sauce
- 1/2 cup roasted peanuts, chopped

Directions:

1. Warm two tablespoons of the sesame oil in a frying pan over medium-high heat. Fry the eggs until they are set or about 5 minutes; reserve.

2. In the same frying pan, heat the remaining tablespoons of sesame oil. Brown, the ground meat, crumbling it with a fork.

3. Add in the ginger-garlic paste, coriander, Chinese cabbage, and onion; continue to cook for a further 6 minutes or until the vegetables have softened.

4. Heat off; stir in the rice wine and hot sauce. Stir to combine well and divide between six plates. Top each serving with a fried egg.

5. Scatter roasted peanuts on the top and serve immediately.

Nutrition:

Calories 538 Fat 41.9g

Carbs 4.9g Protein 34.1g

Fiber 1.6g

Sausage and Cheese Wrap

Preparation Time: 5 Minutes

Cooking Time: 10 Minutes

Servings: 2

Ingredients:

- 2.5 oz grated parmesan cheese

- 1.5 oz grated cheddar cheese
- 1.2 oz sausage, crumbled
- 2 tsp avocado oil

Seasoning:

- 1/3 tsp salt
- 1/8 tsp ground black pepper
- ¼ tsp paprika

Directions:

1. Take a heatproof bowl, place cheese in it, microwave for seconds, stir and microwave for another 10 seconds.
2. Shape the cheese into two balls, place a cheese ball on a parchment sheet, and then cover it with another parchment sheet.
3. Let the cheese cool for 10 seconds, use hands to spread cheese into a circle, and then roll into a thin circle using a rolling pin.
4. Cut extra parchment sheet around the circle, keep cheese tortilla in the refrigerator and repeat with the other cheese ball.
5. Then prepare sausage and for this, take a medium skillet pan, place it over medium heat, add oil and when hot, add sausage, crumble it and cook for 2 minutes until meat begins to brown.
6. Then season it with black pepper, salt, and paprika, stir until mixed and continue cooking for 3 to 4 minutes until cooked.

7. Distribute sausage evenly on prepared cheese tortilla, roll gently, and then serve.

Nutrition:

Calories 461

Fats 38.9 g

Protein 22g

Net Carb 5.8g

Fiber 0g

Broccoli & Ground Beef Casserole

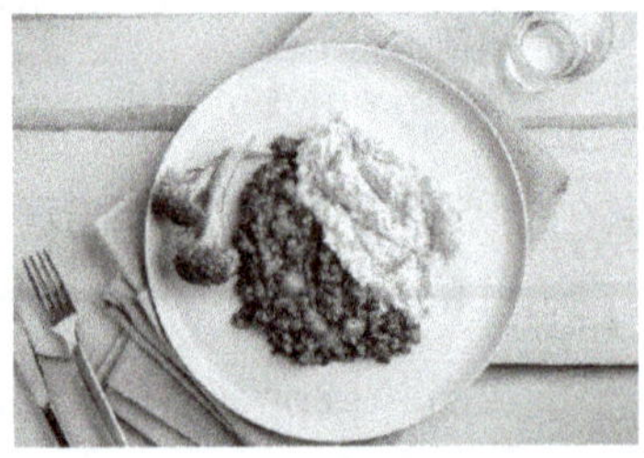

Preparation Time: 5 Minutes

Cooking Time: 4 Hours and 15 Minutes

Servings: 6

Ingredients:

- 1 tbsp olive oil
- 2 pounds ground beef
- One head broccoli, cut into florets
- Salt and black pepper, to taste
- 2 tsp mustard
- 2 tsp Worcestershire sauce
- 28 ounces canned diced tomatoes
- 2 cups mozzarella cheese, grated
- 16 ounces tomato sauce
- 2 tbsp fresh parsley, chopped
- 1 tsp dried oregano

Directions:

1. Apply black pepper and salt to the broccoli florets, set them into a bowl, drizzle over the

olive oil, and toss well to coat completely.

2. In a separate bowl, combine the beef with Worcestershire sauce, salt, mustard, and black pepper, and stir well. Press on the slow cooker's bottom.

3. Scatter in the broccoli, add the tomatoes, parsley, mozzarella, oregano, and tomato sauce. Cook for 4 hours on low; covered.

4. Split the casserole among bowls and enjoy while hot.

Nutrition:

Cal 434

Fat 21g

Net Carbs 5.6g

Protein 51g

Curry Beef

Preparation Time: 5 Minutes

Cooking Time: 30 Minutes

Servings: 4

Ingredients:

- Two shallots, chopped
- Two tablespoons avocado oil
- 1-pound beef stew meat, cubed
- One teaspoon curry powder
- 1 cup beef stock
- 1 cup coconut cream
- A pinch of salt and black pepper
- One tablespoon chive, chopped

Directions:

1. Warm a pan with the oil over medium heat, add the shallots and the

meat, and brown for 5 minutes.

2. Add the curry powder, toss and cook for 5 minutes more.

3. Add the rest of the ingredients, bring to a simmer and cook over medium heat for 20 minutes more, stirring often.

4. Divide the mix into bowls and serve.

Nutrition:

Calories 325

Fat 18

Fiber 1

Carbs 5.6

Protein 36

Sprouts Stir-fry with Kale, Broccoli, And Beef

Preparation Time: 5 Minutes

Cooking Time: 8 Minutes

Servings: 2

Ingredients:

- Three slices of beef roast, chopped
- 2 oz Brussels sprouts, halved
- 4 oz broccoli florets
- 3 oz kale
- 1 ½ tbsp butter, unsalted
- 1/8 tsp red pepper flakes

Seasoning:

- ¼ tsp garlic powder
- ¼ tsp salt
- 1/8 tsp ground black pepper

Directions:

1. Take a medium skillet pan, place it over medium heat, add ¾ tbsp butter and when it melts, add broccoli florets and sprouts, sprinkle with garlic powder, and cook for 2 minutes.

2. Season vegetables with salt and red pepper flakes, add chopped beef, stir until mixed and continue cooking for 3 minutes until browned on one side.

3. Then add kale and remaining butter, flip the vegetables and cook for 2 minutes until kale leaves wilts.

4. Serve.

Nutrition:

Calories 125 Fats 9.4 g Protein 4.8g Net Carb 1.7 g Fiber 2.6g

Korean Braised Beef with Kelp Noodles

Preparation Time: 5 Minutes

Cooking Time: 2 Hours and 15 Minutes

Servings: 4

Ingredients:

- 1 ½ lb. sirloin steak, cut into strips
- 2 (16- oz) packs kelp noodles, thoroughly rinsed
- 1 tbsp coconut oil
- Two pieces star anise
- One cinnamon stick
- One garlic clove, minced
- 1-inch ginger, grated
- 3 tbsp coconut aminos

- 2 tbsp swerve brown sugar
- ¼ cup red wine
- 4 cups beef broth
- One head napa cabbage, steamed
- Scallions, thinly sliced

Directions:

1. Heat oil in a pot over and sauté anise, cinnamon, garlic, and ginger until fragrant, 5 minutes. Add in beef, season with salt and pepper, and sear on both sides
2. In a bowl, combine aminos, sugar, wine, and ¼ cup water. Pour the mixture into the pot, close the lid, and bring to a boil.
3. Lessen the heat and simmer for 1 to 1 ½ hour or until the meat is tender.
4. Strain the pot's content through a colander into a bowl and pour the braising liquid back into the pot.
5. Discard cinnamon and anise and set aside.
6. Add broth and simmer until hot, 10 minutes.
7. Put kelp noodles in the broth and cook until softened and separated, 6 minutes.
8. Spoon the noodles and some broth into bowls, add beef strips, and top with cabbage and scallions.

Nutrition:

Cal 548 Net Carbs 26.6g

Fat 27g Protein 44g

Assorted Grilled Veggies & Beef Steaks

Preparation Time: 5 Minutes

Cooking Time: 30 Minutes

Servings: 4

Ingredients:

- One red and one green bell peppers, cut into strips
- 4 tbsp olive oil
- One ¼ pound sirloin steaks
- Salt and black pepper to taste
- 3 tbsp balsamic vinegar
- ½ lb. asparagus, trimmed
- One eggplant, sliced
- Two zucchinis, sliced
- One red onion, sliced

Directions:

1. Divide the meat and vegetables between 2 bowls.
2. Mix the salt, pepper, olive oil, and balsamic vinegar in a two bowl.
3. Rub the beef all over with half of this mixture.
4. Pour the remaining mixture over the vegetables—Preheat a grill pan.
5. Drain the steaks and reserve the marinade. Sear the steaks on both sides for minutes, flipping once halfway through; set aside.
6. Pour the vegetables and marinade in the pan; and cook for 5 minutes, turning once. Serve.

Nutrition:

Cal 459

Net Carbs 4.5g

Fat 31g

Protein 32.8g

Lemony Sea Bass Fillet

Preparation Time: 10 Minutes

Cooking Time: 15 Minutes

Servings: 4

Ingredients:

Fish:

- Four sea bass fillets
- Two tablespoons olive oil, divided
- A pinch of chili pepper
- Salt, to taste

Olive Sauce:

- One tablespoon green olive, pitted and sliced
- One lemon, juiced
- Salt, to taste

Directions:

1. Preheat the grill to high heat.
2. Stir together one tablespoon olive oil, chili pepper, and salt in a bowl.
3. Brush both sides of each sea bass fillet generously with the mixture.
4. Grill the fillets on the preheated grill for about 5 to 6 minutes on each side until lightly browned.
5. Meanwhile, warm the left olive oil in a skillet over medium heat.
6. Add the green olives, lemon juice, and salt.
7. Cook until the sauce is heated through.

8. Transfer the fillets to four serving plates, then pour the sauce over them. Serve warm.

Nutrition:

Calories: 257

Fat: 12.4g

Fiber: 56.g

Carbohydrates:2 g

Protein: 12.7g

Curried Fish with Super Greens

Preparation Time: 10 Minutes

Cooking Time: 20 Minutes

Servings: 4

Ingredients:

- Two tablespoons coconut oil
- Two teaspoons garlic, minced
- 11/2 tablespoons grated fresh ginger
- 1/2 teaspoon ground cumin
- One tablespoon curry powder
- 2 cups of coconut milk
- 16 ounces (454 g) firm white fish, cut into 1-inch chunks
- 1 cup kale, shredded
- Two tablespoons cilantro, chopped

Directions:

1. Melt the coconut oil in a heated pan
2. Add the garlic and ginger and sauté for about 2 minutes until tender.
3. Fold in the cumin and curry powder, then cook for 1 to 2 minutes until fragrant.

4. Put in the coconut milk and boil. Boil then simmer until the flavors mellow, about 5 minutes.

5. Add the fish chunks and simmer for 10 minutes until the fish flakes easily with a fork, stirring once.

6. Scatter the shredded kale and chopped cilantro over the fish, then cook for 2 minutes more until softened.

Nutrition:

Calories: 376

Fat: 19.9g

Fiber: 15.8g

Carbohydrates: 6.7 g

Protein: 14.8 g

Shrimp Alfredo

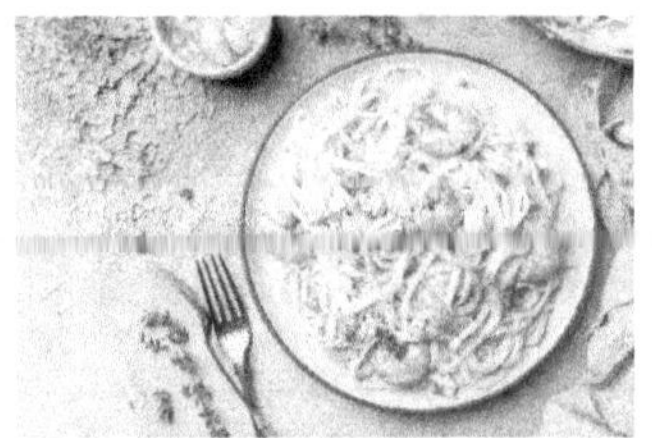

Preparation Time: 15 Minutes

Cooking Time: 30 Minutes

Servings: 4

Ingredients:

- 1 pound of wild shrimp
- Three tablespoons of organic grass-fed whey
- 1 1/2 cups of frozen asparagus
- 1 cup of heavy cream
- 1/2 cup of parmesan cheese
- Sea salt
- Black pepper
- Two ground garlic cloves
- One small diced onion

Directions:

1. Peel and devein the shrimps, coat them well with salt and pepper. Let it cover in a bowl for 20 minutes.
2. Preheat a skillet. Put in butter, garlic, and onions.
3. When butter is melted, put in shrimp and stir fry till for 3 minutes.
4. Pour in heavy cream and stir well. Then, add ion cheese and stir till cheese melts.
5. Serve hot.

Nutrition:

Calories: 315

Fat: 11.9g

Fiber: 8.5g

Carbohydrates:9.3 g

Protein: 11.1g

Garlic-Lemon Mahi Mahi

Preparation Time: 15 Minutes

Cooking Time: 10 Minutes

Servings: 3

Ingredients:

- Six tablespoons of butter
- Five tablespoons of extra-virgin olive oil
- 4 ounces of mahi-mahi fillets
- Three minced cloves of garlic
- Kosher salt
- Black pepper
- 2 pounds of asparagus
- Two sliced lemons
- Zest and juice of 2 lemons
- One teaspoon of crushed red pepper flakes

- One tablespoon of chopped parsley

Directions:

1. Melt three tablespoons of butter and olive oil in a microwave.
2. Heat a skillet and put in mahi-mahi, then sprinkle black pepper.
3. For around 5 minutes per side, cook it. When done, move to a plate.
4. In another skillet, add remaining oil and add in the asparagus, stir fry for 2-3 minutes. Take out on a plate.
5. In the same skillet, pour in the remaining butter, and add garlic, red pepper, lemon, zest, juice, and parsley.
6. Add in the mahi-mahi and asparagus and stir together. Serve hot.

Nutrition:

Calories: 317

Fat: 8.5g

Fiber: 6.9g

Carbohydrates:3.1 g

Protein: 16.1g

Scallops in Creamy Garlic Sauce

Preparation Time: 5 Minutes

Cooking Time: 25 Minutes

Servings: 8

Ingredients:

- 11/4 pounds fresh sea scallops, side muscles removed
- Salt and ground black pepper, as required
- Four tablespoons butter, divided

- Five garlic cloves, chopped
- 1/4 cup homemade chicken broth
- 1 cup heavy cream
- One tablespoon fresh lemon juice
- Two tablespoons fresh parsley, chopped

Directions:

1. Sprinkle the scallops evenly with salt and black pepper.
2. Melt two tablespoons of butter in a large pan over medium-high heat and cook the scallops for about 2–3 minutes per side.
3. Flip the scallops and cook for about two more minutes.
4. With a slotted spoon, transfer the scallops onto a plate.
5. Using the same pan, the butter must be melted and sauté the garlic for about 1 minute.
6. Pour the broth and bring to a gentle boil.
7. Cook for about 2 minutes.
8. Stir in the cream and cook for about 1–2 minutes or until slightly thickened.
9. Stir in the cooked scallops and lemon juice and remove from heat.
10. Garnish with fresh parsley and serve hot.

Nutrition:

Calories: 259

Fat: 8.5g

Fiber: 7.4g

Carbohydrates:2.1 g

Protein: 12.2g

Shrimp Curry

Preparation Time: 15 Minutes

Cooking Time: 20 Minutes

Servings: 4

Ingredients:

- Two tablespoons coconut oil
- 1/2 of yellow onion, minced
- Two garlic cloves, minced
- One teaspoon ground turmeric
- One teaspoon ground cumin
- One teaspoon paprika
- 1 (14-ounce) can unsweetened coconut milk
- One large tomato, chopped finely
- Salt, as required
- 1-pound shrimp, peeled and deveined
- Two tablespoons fresh cilantro, chopped

Directions:

1. The coconut oil must be melted in a wok on medium heat and sauté the onion for about 5 minutes.
2. Add the garlic and spices, and sauté for about 1 minute.
3. Add the coconut milk, tomato, and salt, and bring to a gentle boil.
4. Let the curry simmer for about 10 minutes, stirring occasionally.
5. Stir in the shrimp and cilantro and simmer for about 4–5 minutes.

Nutrition:

Calories: 354

Fat: 12.5g

Fiber:7.5 g

Carbohydrates:4.1 g

Protein: 14.1g

Israeli Salmon Salad

Preparation Time: 10 Minutes

Cooking Time: 0 Minutes

Servings: 2

Ingredients:

- 1 cup flaked smoked salmon
- One tomato, chopped
- 1/2 small red onion, chopped
- One cucumber, chopped
- 6 tbsp. pitted green olives
- One avocado, chopped
- 2 tbsp. avocado oil
- 2 tbsp. almond oil
- 1 tbsp. plain vinegar
- Salt and black pepper to taste
- 1 cup crumbled feta cheese
- 1 cup grated cheddar cheese

Directions:

1. In a salad bowl, add the salmon, tomatoes, red onion, cucumber, green olives, and avocado. Mix well.
2. In a bowl, whisk the avocado oil, vinegar, salt, and black pepper.
3. Drizzle the dressing over the salad and toss well.
4. Sprinkle some feta cheese and serve the salad immediately.

Nutrition:

Calories: 415

Fat: 11.4g

Fiber: 9.9g

Carbohydrates:3.8 g

Protein: 15.4g

Blackened Salmon with Avocado Salsa

Preparation Time: 15 Minutes

Cooking Time: 10 Minutes

Servings: 4

Ingredients:

- 1 tbsp. extra virgin olive oil
- Four filets of salmon (about 6 oz. each)
- 4 tsp. Cajun seasoning
- Two medium avocados, diced
- 1 c. cucumber, diced
- 1/4 c. red onion, diced
- 1 tbsp. parsley, chopped
- 1 tbsp. lime juice
- Sea salt & pepper, to taste

Directions:

1. The oil must be heated in a skillet.
2. Rub the Cajun seasoning into the fillets, then lay them into the bottom of the skillet once it's hot enough.
3. Cook until a dark crust forms, then flip and repeat.
4. In a medium mixing bowl, combine all the ingredients for the salsa and set aside.
5. Plate the fillets and top with 1/4 of the salsa yielded.

6. Enjoy!

Nutrition:

Calories: 425

Fat: 15.8g

Fiber: 19.2g

Carbohydrates:4.1 g

Protein: 11/8g

Tangy Coconut Cod

Preparation Time: 10 Minutes

Cooking Time: 10 Minutes

Servings: 2

Ingredients:

- 1/3 c. coconut flour
- 1/2 tsp. cayenne pepper
- One egg, beaten
- One lime
- 1 tsp. crushed red pepper flakes
- 1 tsp. garlic powder
- 12 oz. cod fillets
- Sea salt & pepper, to taste

Directions:

1. Let the oven preheat to 400°F/175°C. then line a baking sheet with non-stick foil.
2. Place the flour in a shallow dish (a plate works fine) and drag the fillets of cod through the beaten egg. Dredge the cod in the coconut flour, then lay on the baking sheet.
3. Sprinkle the fillet's top with the seasoning and lime juice.
4. Bake the cod for about 10 to 12 minutes until the fillets are flaky.
5. Serve immediately!

Nutrition:

Calories: 318

Fat: 12.1g

Fiber: 15.1g

Carbohydrates:4.1 g

Protein: 19.5g

Fish Taco Bowl

Preparation Time: 10 Minutes

Cooking Time: 15 Minutes

Servings: 2

Ingredients:

- 2 (5-ounce) tilapia fillets
- One tablespoon olive oil
- Four teaspoons Tajin seasoning salt, divided
- 2 cups pre-sliced coleslaw cabbage mix
- One tablespoon avocado mayo
- 1 tsp. hot sauce
- One avocado, mashed
- Pink Himalayan salt
- Freshly ground black pepper

Directions:

1. Preheat the oven to 425 F. The baking sheet must be lined with a baking mat.
2. Rub the tilapia with the olive oil, and then coat it with Tajín seasoning salt with two teaspoons.
3. Place the fish in the prepared pan.
4. Let the tilapia bake for 15 minutes, or until the fish is opaque when you pierce it with a fork.
5. Meanwhile, in a medium bowl, gently mix to combine the coleslaw and the mayo sauce.

6. You don't want the cabbage super wet, just enough to dress it.

7. Add the mashed avocado and the remaining two teaspoons of Tajín seasoning salt to the coleslaw, and season with pink Himalayan salt and pepper.

8. Divide the salad between two bowls.

9. Shred fish into tiny pieces, and add it to the bowls.

10. Top the fish with a drizzle of mayo sauce and serve.

Nutrition:

Calories: 231 Fat: 12.1g

Fiber: 10.3g

Carbohydrates:2.1 g

Protein: 17.3g

Cajun Lobster Tails

Preparation Time: 10 Minutes

Cooking Time: 20 Minutes

Servings: 4

Ingredients:

- 1 lb. of peeled and deveined raw Lobster
- 1 Cup of almond flour
- 1 tbsp. of pepper
- 1 tbsp. of salt
- 1 tsp. of cayenne pepper
- 1 tsp. of cumin
- 1 tsp. of garlic powder
- 1 tbsp. of paprika
- 1 tbsp. of onion powder

Directions:

1. Preheat your fryer to a temperature of 390° F. Peel the lobster and devein it.

2. Dip the lobster into the heavy cream.

3. Dredge the lobster into the mixture of the almond flour. Shake off any excess flour.

4. Put the lobster in the fryer and cook for about 15 minutes and the temperature to 200° C/400° F.

5. You can check your appetizer after about 6 minutes, and you can flip the lobster if needed. Serve and enjoy your lobsters!

Nutrition:

Calories: 321

Fat: 14.1g

Fiber: 12.1g

Carbohydrates: 3.2g

Protein: 8.5g

Spicy Shrimp Skewers

Preparation Time: 5 Minutes

Cooking Time: 9 Minutes

Servings: 4

Ingredients:

- 2 tbsp. Paprika
- 1/2 tbsp. Onion powder
- 1/2 tbsp. dried thyme, crushed
- 1-pound shrimp, peeled and deveined
- 2 tbsp. Olive oil
- 1/2 tbsp. Red chili powder
- 1/2 tbsp. Garlic powder
- 1/2 tbsp. dried oregano, crushed
- Two zucchinis, cut into 1/2-inch cubes

Directions:

1. Preheat the grill to medium-high heat.

2. In a bowl, mix spices and dried herbs.

3. In a large bowl, add shrimp, zucchini, oil, and seasoning and toss to coat well.

4. Thread shrimp and zucchini onto pre-soaked skewers.

5. Grill the skewers for about 6-8 minutes, flipping occasionally. Serve hot.

Nutrition:

Calories: 261

Fat: 9.4g

Fiber: 10.1g

Carbohydrates:3.2 g

Protein: 4.1g

Crack Slaw

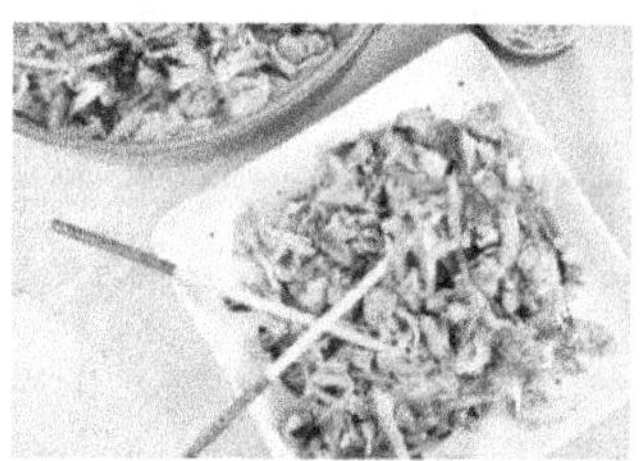

Preparation Time: 5 Minutes

Cooking Time: 35 Minutes

Servings: 4

Ingredients:

- Two tablespoons butter, ghee, or coconut oil

- 1-pound ground pork or sausage

- One small head of green cabbage, shredded

- Two tablespoons liquid or coconut aminos

- One tablespoon fish sauce

- One tablespoon coconut vinegar or apple cider vinegar

- One teaspoon garlic powder
- One teaspoon onion powder
- ¼ teaspoon ground ginger
- Pinch red pepper flakes
- Pinch sea salt
- Pinch freshly ground black pepper
- One scallion, chopped

Directions:

1. In a large skillet over medium heat, melt the butter or heat the oil and add the ground pork or sausage. Cook, stirring, until browned, 5 to 7 minutes.
2. Add the shredded cabbage and mix to combine. Add the aminos, fish sauce, vinegar, garlic powder, onion powder, ginger, and red pepper flakes and mix well.
3. Simmer on low for 20 to 30 minutes, occasionally stirring, until the cabbage is cooked down and tender.
4. Season with salt and pepper and top with the chopped scallion.
5. Serve immediately or store in the refrigerator for up to 1 week.

Nutrition:

Calories: 356

Total Fat: 24g

Protein: 24g

Total Carbs: 11g

Slow Cooker Pulled Pork

Preparation Time: 5 Minutes

Cooking Time: 8 to 10 Hours

Servings: 12

Ingredients:

- One large onion, sliced
- Six garlic cloves smashed
- One tablespoon ground cumin
- One tablespoon chili powder
- Two teaspoons sea salt
- One teaspoon freshly ground black pepper
- ½ teaspoon cayenne pepper (optional)
- 1 (4- to 6-pound) boneless pork shoulder (or 6 to 8 pounds bone-in)
- 2 cups Bone Broth

Directions:

1. Arrange the onion slices on the bottom of the slow cooker and scatter the garlic cloves over the top.

2. In a small bowl, whisk together the cumin, chili powder, salt, pepper, and cayenne (if using). Rub the spice mixture all over the pork shoulder. Place the meat on top of the onion and garlic in the slow cooker.

3. Pour the bone broth over the pork, cover, and cook on high for 2 hours. Reduce the heat to low and cook for another 6 hours until the meat is tender and falls apart quickly. Do not lift the lid during cooking. Alternatively,

you can cook on low for 8 to 10 hours.

4. Transfer the pork to a bowl, reserving the broth for the sauces, and shred it using two forks.

Nutrition:

Calories: 224

Total Fat: 16g

Protein: 20g

Total Carbs: 0g

Bacon Mac 'N' Cheese

Preparation Time: 10 Minutes

Cooking Time: 20 Minutes

Servings: 6

Ingredients:

- One cauliflower head, chopped into small pieces (about 4 cups)
- Six bacon slices
- ½ cup heavy (whipping) cream
- 3 ounces cream cheese, cut into cubes
- 1½ cups shredded sharp Cheddar cheese
- Two teaspoons Dijon or yellow mustard
- One teaspoon garlic powder
- One teaspoon onion powder
- One teaspoon paprika
- ¼ teaspoon cayenne pepper
- Sea salt
- Freshly ground black pepper
- Chopped fresh parsley (optional)

Directions:

1. In a large microwave-safe dish, cook the

cauliflower florets on high for 15 to 20 minutes until tender. Alternatively, you can steam the cauliflower on the stovetop until tender. If using frozen cauliflower, follow the package instructions for steaming, but be careful not to overcook it.

2. Meanwhile, in a large skillet, cook the bacon over medium-high heat for 5 to 7 minutes until crisp. Transfer to a paper towel and let cool. Reserve the bacon grease for the sauce, if desired.

3. Although the bacon and cauliflower are cooking, prepare the cheese sauce.

4. In a large saucepan over medium-low heat, bring the cream to a simmer.

5. Add the cream cheese, then cook, beating until the cream cheese melts.

6. Add the Cheddar, garlic powder, mustard, onion powder, paprika, and cayenne. Lessen the heat to low and cook, whisking, until the Cheddar melts. Remain to cook on low heat, continually whisking, for 2 to 3 minutes more until the sauce thickens.

7. Take away the pan from the heat and season with salt and pepper. The sauce will be thick, but it will thin out a bit once you add the cauliflower.

8. Drain any extra liquid from the cauliflower

and stirring it into the cheese sauce. Smash in the bacon and stir to combine.

9. Serve immediately, garnished with parsley.

Nutrition:

Calories: 307

Total Fat: 25g

Protein: 13g

Total Carbs: 7.5g

Pork Tenderloin with Creamy Horseradish Sauce

Preparation Time: 5 Minutes

Cooking Time: 25 Minutes

Servings: 4

Ingredients:

- One pork tenderloin (about 1 pound)
- One teaspoon garlic powder
- One teaspoon onion powder
- One teaspoon sea salt
- ½ teaspoon freshly ground black pepper
- One tablespoon avocado or coconut oil or lard
- ½ *cup* Bone Broth
- Two tablespoons butter or ghee
- Two tablespoons heavy (whipping) cream
- One tablespoon Dijon mustard
- One tablespoon spicy horseradish
- ¼ teaspoon cayenne pepper
- One teaspoon gelatin or 1/8 teaspoon xanthan or guar gum to thicken (optional)

Directions:

1. Season the pork by means of the garlic powder, onion powder, pepper, and salt

2. In a large frypan, heat the oil or lard over medium-high heat.

3. Add the pork and brown for 3 to 4 minutes on one side. Rotate the pork one-third of the way and brown for another 3 to 4 minutes. Do it again for the last side.

4. Take away the pork to a plate to rest. It will not be prepared all the way through yet, which is okay because it will cook more in the sauce.

5. Put the skillet back on the stove over medium-high heat.

6. Add the bone broth and boil, scraping the drippings and brown bits off the skillet's bottom.

7. Lessen the heat to medium and whisk in the butter, cream, mustard, horseradish, cayenne, and gelatin. Let simmer, often whisking, for 5 minutes.

8. Once the sauce starts to thicken, cut the pork into ½-inch-thick pieces, and put them back in the skillet. Coat the meat with the sauce, then simmer for another 5 minutes until the pork is cooked through.

Nutrition:

Calories: 243 Total Fat: 15g

Protein: 25g Total Carbs: 2g

Chesos (Cheese Shell Tacos) Carnitas

Preparation Time: 10 Minutes

Cooking Time: 10 Minutes

Servings: 4

Ingredients:

- 2 cups shredded Cheddar cheese
- 2 cups Slow Cooker Pulled Pork
- Two tablespoons Mexican Spice Blend

Topping Suggestions

- Avocado slices
- Sour cream
- Salsa
- Jalapeños
- Chopped onion
- Fresh cilantro
- Hot sauce

Directions:

1. Preheat the oven to 400 F.

2. Put ¼-cup piles of shredded cheese on the prepared baking sheet, forming them into even circles. Consent several inches between the piles to ensure the cheese shells don't melt together.

3. Bake for 6 to 8 minutes or wait until the cheese melts and the edges are lightly browned.

4. Wrap the handle of two wooden spoons or skewers by aluminum foil and balance each one between two cans or cups.

5. Take away the cheese from the oven and let cool for 3 minutes. By means of a spatula,

drape each cheese round over one of the skewers or foil handles. The cheese will roughen into a shell shape as it sets, about 10 minutes.

6. Whereas the chesos are hardening, toss the pork in the Mexican spice blend and warm it in the microwave or oven.

7. Put each cheese shell with ¼ cup of pork and add your anticipated toppings.

Nutrition:

Calories: 385

Total Fat: 29g

Protein: 28g

Total Carbs: 3g

Pork Fried Cauliflower Rice

Preparation Time: 10 Minutes

Cooking Time: 20 Minutes

Servings: 4

Ingredients:

- 1-pound ground pork
- Sea salt
- Freshly ground black pepper
- Three tablespoons toasted sesame oil
- 3 cups thinly sliced cabbage
- 1 cup chopped broccoli
- One red bell pepper, cored and chopped
- One garlic clove, minced
- 1½ cups riced cauliflower
- One tablespoon sriracha

- Two tablespoons liquid aminos or tamari
- One teaspoon rice wine vinegar
- One teaspoon sesame seed, for garnish

Directions:

1. Heat a medium skillet over medium-high heat. Put the pork and sprinkle generously with salt and pepper. Cook, frequently stirring, until browned, about 10 minutes. Take away the meat from the skillet.

2. Lessen the heat to medium and add the sesame oil to the skillet and cabbage, broccoli, bell pepper, riced cauliflower, and garlic. Cook for about 5 minutes until somewhat softened, then add the sriracha, liquid aminos, and vinegar and mix well.

3. Put the browned pork back in the skillet. Simmer together for around 5 minutes more until the cabbage is tender.

4. Season with salt and pepper, then garnish with the sesame seeds and serve right away.

Nutrition:

Calories: 460

Total Fat: 36g

Protein: 23g

Total Carbs: 11g

Lemon Butter Pork Chops

Preparation Time: 5 Minutes

Cooking Time: 25 Minutes

Servings: 4

Ingredients:

- ½ teaspoon of sea salt
- One teaspoon lemon-pepper seasoning
- One teaspoon garlic powder
- ½ teaspoon dried thyme
- 4 (4-ounce) boneless pork chops
- Five tablespoons butter, divided
- ¼ *cup* Bone Broth
- Two tablespoons freshly squeezed lemon juice
- One tablespoon minced garlic
- ½ cup heavy (whipping) cream

Directions:

1. In a small bowl, stir the salt, lemon-pepper seasoning, garlic powder, and thyme.
2. Rub the spice combination all over the pork chops.
3. Heat a frypan over medium-high heat and melt two tablespoons of butter. Add the pork chops and cook for around 5 minutes on each side until they are cooked through. Take away the chops from the pan.
4. Lessen the heat to medium-low. Put the bone broth, lemon juice, garlic, and the remaining three

tablespoons of butter. Add the pork chops and cook for about 15 minutes, adding the cream one tablespoon at a time every few minutes, until the sauce thickens.

5. Remove from the heat and serve.

Nutrition:

Calories: 379 Total Fat: 29g

Protein: 27g Total Carbs: 2.5g

Creamy Pork Marsala

Preparation Time: 5 Minutes

Cooking Time: 30 Minutes

Servings: 4

Ingredients:

- 4 (4-ounce) boneless pork cutlets
- Salt
- Freshly ground black pepper
- Four tablespoons butter
- 8 ounces sliced mushrooms
- 4 ounces prosciutto, chopped
- One garlic clove, minced
- ½ cup Marsala cooking wine
- *½ cup* Bone Broth
- One teaspoon chopped fresh thyme
- ½ teaspoon xanthan or guar gum,
- Chopped fresh parsley for garnish

Directions:

1. Sprinkle the cutlets with pepper and salt.

2. Heat a large frypan with medium-high heat and melt two tablespoons of

butter. Add the cutlets, then cook for at least 5 minutes on each side until cooked completely. Take away the cutlets from the skillet.

3. Lessen the heat to medium-low and add the remaining two tablespoons of butter. Add the mushrooms, prosciutto, garlic, and cook, frequently stirring, until the mushrooms brown, about 5 minutes.

4. Add the wine, bone broth, and thyme.

5. Cook for around 15 minutes until the sauce thickens. Add the xanthan gum to thicken the sauce even more. Put the pork back in the skillet and raise the heat to medium-high. Cook until the cutlets are heated through.

6. Serve garnished with parsley.

Nutrition:

Calories: 339

Total Fat: 19g

Protein: 36g

Total Carbs: 6g

CHAPTER 8:

Snacks

Chocolate Cupcakes

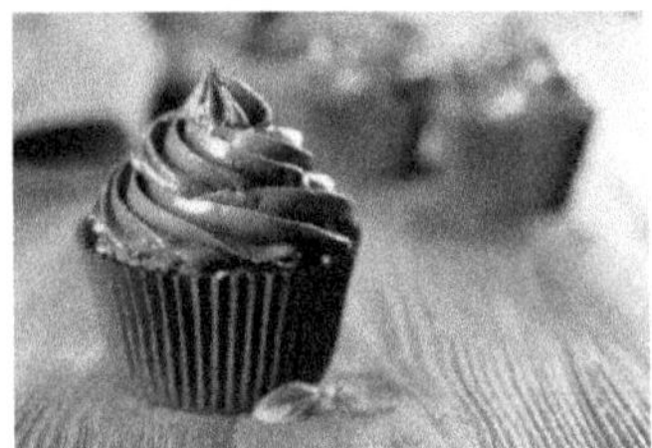

Preparation Time: 5 Minutes

Cooking Time: 20 Minutes

Servings: 6

Ingredients:

- 1 ½ cups of almond flour
- 1 cup shredded coconut
- Two large eggs
- ¼ cup cream cheese
- 3 tbsp plain Greek yogurt
- ¼ cup swerve

- 2 tbsp cocoa powder, unsweetened
- 3 tbsp butter
- 2 tsp baking powder
- Spices:
- 1 tsp vanilla extract

Directions:

1. In a large mixing bowl, place eggs and butter. Beat well on high speed until light and fluffy mixture. Then add swerve, cream cheese, and Greek yogurt. Continue to mix until smooth.
2. Finally, add almond flour, shredded coconut, and baking powder. Mix well.

3. Divide the mixture between 6 silicone cups and set aside.

4. Plugin the instant pot and position a trivet at the bottom of the inner pot. Pour in 1 cup of water and carefully place cups on the trivet.

5. Put the timer for 10 minutes on the "Manual" mode.

6. Perform a rapid pressure release and open the lid. Remove the cups from the pot and cool to room temperature.

Nutrition:

Calories 212

Total Fats: 18.9g

Carbs: 4.2g

Protein: 6g

Chocolate Chip Mug Cake

Preparation Time: 5 Minutes

Cooking Time: 10 Minutes

Servings: 1

Ingredients:

- 3 tbsp almond flour
- 3 tbsp coconut oil, softened
- 1 tbsp cocoa powder, unsweetened
- 1 tbsp chocolate chips, unsweetened
- ½ tsp baking powder
- 2 tsp swerve

Spices:

- ¼ tsp vanilla extract

Directions:

1. In a small bowl, combine the ingredients and mix well until fully incorporated. Transfer

the mixture to an oven-safe mug and loosely cover with aluminum foil

2. Plugin the instant pot, then pour in one cup of water.

3. Place a trivet at the bottom of the inner pot and place the mug on top.

4. Press the "Manual" button and set the timer for 5 minutes on high pressure.

5. When done, perform a quick pressure release and open the lid. Cool for a while and serve.

Nutrition:

Calories 464

Total Fats: 48g

Carbs: 9.1g

Protein: 3.3g

Creamy Coconut Hazelnut Cake

Preparation Time: 5 Minutes

Cooking Time: 35 Minutes

Servings: 10

Ingredients:

- 2 cups coconut flour
- ¼ cup almond flour
- 3 tbsp shredded coconut
- 3 tsp baking powder
- 1 cup coconut cream
- Five large eggs
- ¼ cup erythritol
- 2 cups whipping cream, sugar-free
- 3 tbsp hazelnuts, finely chopped

Spices:

- 2 tsp vanilla extract

Directions:

1. Plugin the instant pot and pour in one cup of water. Place a trivet at the bottom of the inner pot, then set aside,

2. In a large mixing bowl, combine all dry fixings and mix well.

3. Put eggs, one at a time, then beat well on medium-high speed.

4. Now add coconut cream and vanilla extract. Continue to beat for two more minutes on medium speediness

5. Grease a small pan with some coconut oil and pour in the mixture.

6. In the pot, place the mixture and seal the lid.

7. Next, you need to set the steam release handle, then press the "Manual" button.

8. Set the timer for 20 minutes on high pressure.

9. Beat the whipping cream and wait until light and fluffy.

10. Add chopped hazelnuts and optionally some finely chopped almonds.

11. Refrigerate until use.

12. When you hear the cooker's end signal, perform a quick pressure release, and open the lid. Remove the pan from the pot and cool for a while.

13. Top with whipped cream and refrigerate for 2-3 hours before serving.

Nutrition:

Calories 217

Total Fats: 18.2g

Carbs: 5.1g

Protein: 5.8g

Ice Cream Brownies

Preparation Time: 5 Minutes

Cooking Time: 40 Minutes

Servings: 6

Ingredients:

For the brownies:

- 1 cup almond flour
- ¼ cup coconut flour
- ¼ cup shredded coconut
- 1 tsp baking powder
- Three large eggs
- ¼ cup butter, melted
- 3 tbsp granulated stevia

For the ice cream:

- 1 cup plain Greek yogurt
- ¼ cup whipping cream
- ½ tsp agar powder
- 1 tbsp lemon zest
- 2 tsp vanilla extract
- ¼ cup swerve

Directions:

1. In a large mixing bowl, put Greek yogurt, whipping cream, agar powder, lemon zest, vanilla extract, and swerve. With a paddle attachment on, beat well on medium-high speed until light and fluffy. Transfer to the refrigerator and set aside.

2. Now, prepare the brownies. Combine all dry ingredients and mix

well. Put eggs, one at a time, then beat well with a paddle attachment on. Pour in the melted butter and continue to beat until fully incorporated.

3. Line a small cake pans with some parchment paper and adds the brownie mixture. Using a kitchen spatula, flatten the surface as evenly as possible and tightly wrap with aluminum foil.

4. Plugin the instant pot and pour in 1 cup of water. Set the trivet and add the cake pan.

5. Cook for 15 minutes on high pressure.

6. When done, perform a quick pressure release and open the lid.

7. Cautiously remove the pan from the pot and cool it to room temperature.

8. Top with the ice cream mixture and refrigerate for about an hour.

Nutrition:

Calories 174

Total Fats: 14.2g

Net Carbs: 3.3g

Protein: 5.3g

Mint Brownies with Hazelnuts

Preparation Time: 5 Minutes

Cooking Time: 35 Minutes

Servings: 6

Ingredients:

- ¾ cup almond flour
- ½ cup flaxseed meal

- ½ cup Mascarpone
- Four large eggs
- 2 tbsp butter
- ¼ cup swerve
- 3 tbsp hazelnuts, finely chopped
- Spices:
- ¼ tsp salt
- 1 tsp mint extract

Directions:

1. Combine the fixings in a large mixing bowl and beat well on medium speed until fully incorporated and smooth.
2. Line a small cake pans with parchment paper and brush with some oil. Pour in the batter and loosely cover with aluminum foil.
3. Plugin the instant pot and set the trivet in the inner pot. Pour in approximately one cup of water and place the cake pan on top.
4. Seal the lid and set the steam release grip to the "Sealing" position. Press the "Manual" button and set the timer for 25 minutes.
5. When completed, perform a rapid pressure release and open the lid. Prudently remove the pan from the pot and chill for a while.
6. Slice into eight brownies and serve.

Nutrition:

Calories 203

Total Fats: 15.8g

Net Carbs: 1.6g

Protein: 9.4g

Mocha Pots de Creme

Preparation Time: 5 Minutes

Cooking Time: 25 Minutes

Servings: 4

Ingredients:

- Two large eggs, separated
- 1 cup milk, full-fat
- ¾ cup heavy cream
- 3 tbsp stevia powder
- 2 tbsp cocoa powder, unsweetened
- 3 tbsp brewed espresso

Spices:

- ¼ tsp salt
- 1 tsp vanilla extract

Directions:

1. Put eggs, cocoa powder, espresso, stevia powder, vanilla, and salt. Set aside.
2. Plugin the instant pot and press the "Sauté" button. Pour in the milk and heavy cream. Give it a good stir and warm up.
3. Press the "Cancel" button, then gradually pour the warm milk mixture over the egg mixture, whisking constantly.
4. Divide the mixture between 4 ramekins and loosely cover with aluminum foil.
5. Arrange a trivet at the bottom of your pot and pour in 2 cups of water. Gently place the ramekins on top and seal the lid.
6. Put the steam release handle to the "Sealing" position and press the "Manual" button.

7. Cook for 15 minutes.

8. When done, perform a quick pressure release and open the lid. Remove the ramekins and transfer them to a wire rack. Cool to room temperature and then refrigerate for about an hour.

Nutrition:

Calories 257

Total Fats: 25.5g

Net Carbs: 3.5g

Protein: 5.5g

Chocolate Chip Pudding

Preparation Time: 5 Minutes

Cooking Time: 15 Minutes

Servings: 4

Ingredients:

- 1 cup unsweetened almond milk
- ¼ cup swerve
- 1 tbsp agar powder
- ¼ cup almonds, finely chopped
- 2 tbsp cocoa powder, unsweetened
- 2 tbsp chocolate chips, sugar-free
- One ¼ cup whipping cream
- ½ cup coconut cream
- Spices:
- 1 tsp vanilla extract

Directions:

1. Plugin the instant pot and pour in the milk. Press the "Sauté" button and heat up. Add swerve, cocoa powder, coconut cream, and vanilla extract.

2. Bring it to a boil, stirring constantly, and then add agar powder. Continue to cook for 1-2 minutes.

3. Press the "Cancel" button and stir in finely chopped almonds.

4. Transfer the combination to a large mixing bowl and pour in the whipping cream. Beat well at high speed for 2-3 minutes.

5. Finally, divide the mixture between serving bowls and cool completely before serving.

Nutrition:

Calories 257

Total Fats: 24.5g

Net Carbs: 6.5g

Protein: 3.9g

Vanilla Cherry Panna Cotta

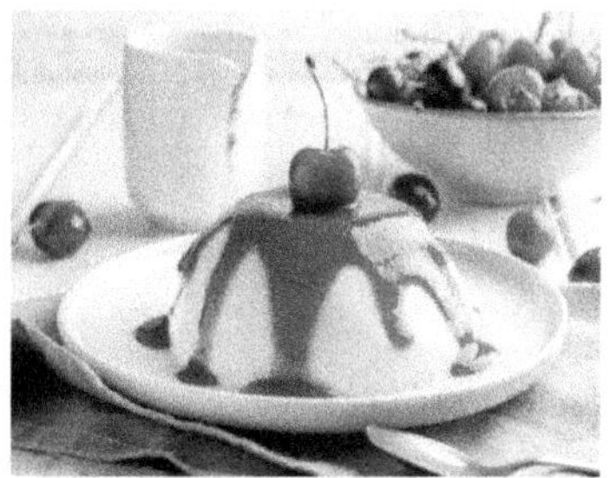

Preparation Time: 5 Minutes

Cooking Time: 15 Minutes

Servings: 2

Ingredients:

For the vanilla layer:

- 1 cup heavy whipping cream
- 2 tbsp whole milk
- 1 tsp agar powder
- ½ tsp vanilla extract
- 1 tbsp walnuts, roughly chopped

For the cherry layer:

- 1 cup heavy whipping cream

- 1 tsp agar powder
- 1 tbsp almonds, roughly chopped
- 2 tsp cherry extract

Directions:

1. Plugin the instant pot and combine all vanilla layer ingredients in the stainless-steel insert. Press the "Sauté" button and stir constantly. Let it simmer and then press the "Cancel" button. Transfer to a large bowl and set aside.
2. Clean the pot and pat dry with kitchen paper.
3. Add all cherry layer ingredients and stir well. Again, bring it to a light simmer, stirring constantly.
4. Pour about the ½-inch thick vanilla layer in a medium-sized glass.
5. Now, pour the second layer of the cherry combination. Do the process again until you have used both mixtures.
6. Garnish with some fresh mint and refrigerate for at least 1 hour before serving.
7. Enjoy!

Nutrition:

Calories 467

Total Fats: 48.7g

Net Carbs: 4.6g

Protein: 4.5g

Orange Lime Pudding

Preparation Time: 5 Minutes

Cooking Time: 10 Minutes

Servings: 4

Ingredients:

- ¼ cup almond milk, unsweetened
- 1 tsp agar powder
- ¼ cup coconut cream
- ¼ cup whipping cream
- 1 tbsp stevia powder
- 1 tbsp coconut oil

Spices:

- 1 tsp orange extract
- 1 tsp lime zest, freshly grated

Directions:

1. Plugin your instant pot and place coconut oil in the stainless-steel insert. Press the "Sauté" button and gently stir with a wooden spatula.

2. When melted, add almond milk, coconut cream, and whipping cream. Bring it to a light simmer, stirring continually.

3. Stir in the stevia powder, agar powder, and orange extract. Cook for another 2-3 minutes, stirring constantly.

4. Turn off the pot and pour the pudding into serving bowls or ramekins immediately.

5. Let it cool to room temperature. Sprinkle with lime zest and refrigerate for 1 hour before serving.

6. Enjoy!

Nutrition:

Calories 155

Total Fats: 12.3g

Net Carbs: 10.7

Protein: 0.7g

Guacamole Deviled Eggs

Preparation Time: 15 Minutes

Cooking Time: 0 Minutes

Servings: 4

Ingredients:

- Eight large eggs
- ½ cup chopped avocado
- Two tablespoons canned coconut milk
- One tablespoon chopped cilantro
- One teaspoon fresh lime juice
- ¼ teaspoon ground cumin
- Salt and pepper to taste
- Paprika for garnish

Directions:

1. Put the eggs in a pan, then cover with water.
2. Bring the water to a boil, then remove from heat and let rest for 10 minutes.
3. Rinse the eggs in cold water until cool enough to handle, then peel.
4. Cut the eggs in half and spoon the yolks into a bowl.
5. Add the avocado, coconut milk, cilantro, lime juice, and cumin.
6. Season with pepper and salt, then stir until smooth.

7. Spoon or pipe the mixture into the egg halves, then sprinkle with paprika.

Nutrition:

Calories 185

Fat 15g

Protein 12g

Net Carbs 2g

Curry Spiced Almonds

Preparation Time: 5 Minutes

Cooking Time: 25 Minutes

Servings: 4

Ingredients:

- 1 cup whole almonds
- Two teaspoons olive oil
- 1 teaspoon curry powder
- ¼ teaspoon salt
- ¼ teaspoon ground turmeric
- Pinch cayenne

Directions:

1. Preheat the oven to 300 F
2. In a mixing bowl, whisk the spices and olive oil.
3. Toss in the almonds, then spread on the baking sheet.
4. Bake for 25 minutes until toasted, then cool and store in an airtight container.

Nutrition:

Calories 155

Fat 14g

Protein 5g

Net Carbs 2g

Chia Peanut Butter Bites

Preparation Time: 10 Minutes

Cooking Time: 10 Minutes

Servings: 6

Ingredients:

- ½ ounce of raw almonds
- One tablespoon powdered erythritol
- Four teaspoons coconut oil
- Two tablespoons canned coconut milk
- ½ teaspoon vanilla extract
- Two tablespoons chia seeds, ground to powder
- ¼ cup coconut cream

Directions:

1. Put the almonds in a skillet over medium-low heat, and cook until toasted. Takes about 5 minutes.
2. Transfer the almonds to a food processor with the erythritol and one teaspoon coconut oil.
3. Blend until it forms a smooth almond butter.
4. Heat the rest of the coconut oil in a skillet over medium heat.
5. Add the coconut milk and vanilla and bring to a simmer.
6. Stir in the ground chia seeds, coconut cream, and almond butter.
7. Cook for 2 minutes, then spread in a foil-lined square dish.
8. Chill until the mixture is firm, then cut into squares to serve.

Nutrition: Calories 110

Fat 8g Protein 2g Net Carbs 7g

Cheesy Sausage Dip

Preparation Time: 10 Minutes

Cooking Time: 2 Hours

Servings: 12

Ingredients:

- ½ pound ground Italian sausage
- ½ cup diced tomatoes
- Two green onions, sliced thin
- 4 ounces cream cheese, cubed
- 4 ounces pepper jack cheese, cubed
- 1 cup sour cream

Directions:

1. Brown the sausage in a skillet, wait for it to cook completely, then stir in the tomatoes.
2. Cook for 2 minutes, stirring often, then stir in the green onions.
3. Line the bottom of a slow cooker with the cheeses, then spoon the sausage mixture on top.
4. Spoon the sour cream over the sausage, then cover and cook on high heat for 2 hours, stirring once halfway through.
5. Serve with celery sticks or pork rinds for dipping.

Nutrition:

Calories 170 Fat 15g

Protein 7g Net Carbs 2g

Salted Kale Chips

Preparation Time: 10 Minutes

Cooking Time: 12 Minutes

Servings: 2

Ingredients:

- ½ bunch fresh kale

- 1 tablespoon olive oil
- Salt and pepper to taste

Directions:

1. Preheat the oven to 350 F and line a baking sheet with foil.
2. Fit the thick stems from the kale and then tear the leaves into pieces.
3. Toss the kale with olive oil and spread it on the baking sheet.
4. Bake for 10 to 12 minutes until crisp, then sprinkle with salt and pepper.

Nutrition:

Calories 75

Fat 7g

Protein 1g

Net Carbs 3g

Bacon Jalapeno Quick Bread

Preparation Time: 20 Minutes

Cooking Time: 45 Minutes

Servings: 10

Ingredients:

- Four slices of thick-cut bacon
- Three jalapeno peppers
- ½ cup coconut flour sifted
- ½ teaspoon baking soda
- ½ teaspoon salt
- Six large eggs, beaten
- ½ cup coconut oil, melted
- ¼ cup of water

Directions:

1. Preheat the oven to 400 F
2. Grease a loaf pan with cooking spray.

3. Spread the bacon and jalapenos on a baking sheet and roast for 10 minutes, stirring halfway through.

4. Crumble the bacon and cut the jalapenos in half to remove the seeds.

5. Combine the bacon and jalapeno in a food processor and pulse until well chopped.

6. Beat together the coconut flour, baking soda, and salt in a bowl.

7. Add the eggs, coconut oil, and water, then stir in the bacon and jalapenos.

8. Spread in the loaf pan, then bake for 40 to 45 minutes until a knife inserted in the center comes out clean.

Nutrition:

Calories 225

Fat 19g Protein 8g

Net Carbs 3g

Toasted Pumpkin Seeds

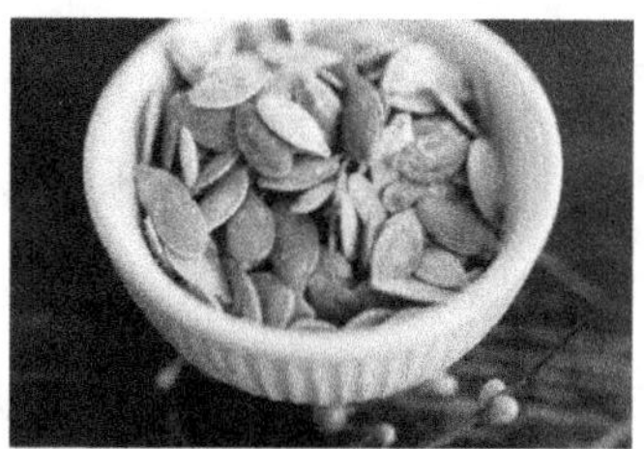

Preparation Time: 5 Minutes

Cooking Time: 5 Minutes

Servings: 2

Ingredients:

- ½ cup hulled pumpkin seeds
- Two teaspoons coconut oil
- Two teaspoons chili powder
- ½ teaspoon salt

Directions:

1. Heat a cast-iron skillet over medium heat.
2. Add the pumpkin seeds and let them cook until toasted, about 3 to 5 minutes, stirring often.
3. Remove from heat and stir in the coconut oil, chili powder, and salt.
4. Let the seeds cool, then store in an airtight container.

Nutrition:

Calories 100 Fat 8.5g

Protein 5.5g Net Carbs 0.5g

Bacon-Wrapped Burger Bites

Preparation Time: 5 Minutes

Cooking Time: 60 Minutes

Servings: 6

Ingredients:

- 6 ounces ground beef (80% lean)
- ¼ teaspoon onion powder
- ¼ teaspoon garlic powder
- ¼ teaspoon ground cumin
- Salt and pepper to taste
- Six slices bacon, uncooked

Directions:

1. Preheat the oven to 350 F
2. Combine the onion powder, garlic powder, cumin, salt, and pepper in a bowl.
3. Add the beef and stir until well combined.
4. Divide the ground beef mixture into six even

portions and roll them into balls.

5. Wrap each ball with a slice of bacon and place it on the baking sheet.

6. Bake for 60 minutes until the bacon is crisp and the beef is cooked through.

Nutrition:

Calories 150

Fat 10g Protein 16g

Net Carbs 0.5g

Almond Sesame Crackers

Preparation Time: 10 Minutes

Cooking Time: 15 Minutes

Servings: 6

Ingredients:

- 1 ½ cups almond flour
- ½ cup sesame seeds
- 1 teaspoon dried oregano
- ½ teaspoon salt
- 1 large egg, whisked
- One tablespoon coconut oil, melted

Directions:

1. Preheat the oven to 350 F

2. Whisk together the almond flour, sesame seeds, oregano, and salt in a bowl.

3. Add the eggs and coconut oil, stirring into a soft dough.

4. Sandwich the dough between two sheets of parchment and roll to 1/8 thickness.

5. Cut into squares and arrange them on the baking sheet.

6. Bake for 10 to 12 minutes or wait until browned around the edges.

Nutrition:

Calories 145

Fat 12.5g

Protein 5g

Net Carbs 2g

Cauliflower Cheese Dip

Preparation Time: 5 Minutes

Cooking Time: 15 Minutes

Servings: 6

Ingredients:

- One small head cauliflower, chopped
- ¾ cup chicken broth
- ¼ teaspoon ground cumin
- ¼ teaspoon chili powder
- ¼ teaspoon garlic powder
- Salt and pepper to taste
- 1/3 cup cream cheese, chopped
- Two tablespoons canned coconut milk

Directions:

1. Combine the cauliflower and chicken broth in a saucepan and simmer until the cauliflower is tender.
2. Add the cumin, chili powder, and garlic powder, then season with salt and pepper.
3. Stir in the cream cheese until melted, then blend everything with an immersion blender.

4. Whisk in the coconut milk, then spoon into a serving bowl.

5. Serve with sliced celery sticks.

Nutrition:

Calories 75

Fat 6g

Protein 2.5g

Net Carbs 2g

Deviled Eggs with Bacon

Preparation Time: 2 Minutes

Cooking Time: 20 Minutes

Servings: 6

Ingredients:

- Six large eggs
- Three slices of thick-cut bacon
- ¼ cup avocado oil mayonnaise
- 1 teaspoon Dijon mustard

Directions:

1. Place the eggs in a saucepan, then pour it with water.

2. Bring the water to boil, then remove from heat and let rest for 10 minutes.

3. Meanwhile, cook the bacon in a skillet over medium-high heat until crisp.

4. Rinse the eggs in cold water until cool enough to handle, then peel them.

5. Cut the eggs in half and spoon the yolks into a bowl.

6. Add one tablespoon of bacon fat from the

skillet along with the mayonnaise and mustard.

7. Spoon the mixture into the egg halves, then crumble the bacon over the top.

Nutrition:

Calories 145 Fat 11g

Protein 8.5g Net Carbs 3g

Coleslaw with Avocado Dressing

Preparation Time: 15 Minutes

Cooking Time: 0 Minutes

Servings: 6

Ingredients:

- One small head green cabbage, sliced thin
- ½ cup shredded red cabbage
- One small red pepper, diced
- 1 cup avocado oil
- 1 large egg, beaten
- Juice from 1 lime
- 1 clove garlic, minced
- Salt to taste

Directions:

1. Combine the shredded cabbages with the red peppers in a bowl.
2. Place the avocado oil, egg, lime juice, and garlic in a blender.
3. Blend smooth, then season with salt to taste.
4. Toss the dressing with the salad and chill until ready to serve.

Nutrition:

Calories 100 Fat, 6g

Protein, 3g

Net Carbs 6g

Creamsicle Fat Bombs

Preparation Time: 5 Minutes

Cooking Time: 0 Minutes

Servings: 10

Ingredients:

- 4 ounces cream cheese, softened
- ½ cup heavy cream
- ½ cup of coconut oil
- One teaspoon orange extract
- 8 to 12 drops liquid stevia extract

Directions:

1. Combine the cream cheese, heavy cream, and coconut oil in a bowl.
2. Blend with an immersion blender until smooth – microwave if needed to soften.
3. Stir in the orange extract and liquid stevia.
4. Spoon the mixture into silicone molds and freeze for 3 hours until solid.
5. Remove the fat bombs from the mold and store them in the freezer.

Nutrition:

Calories 155

Fat 17g

Protein 1g

Net Carbs 0.5g

Baked Cauliflower Bites

Preparation Time: 15 Minutes

Cooking Time: 25 Minutes

Servings: 4

Ingredients:

- One small head cauliflower, chopped

- ¼ cup coconut flour
- Two large eggs
- ½ teaspoon garlic powder
- ¼ teaspoon onion powder
- Salt and pepper to taste

Directions:

1. Preheat the oven to 400 F
2. Place the cauliflower in a saucepan, then cover with water.
3. Boil until the cauliflower is tender, then drain and place in a food processor.
4. Pulse into rice-like grains, then pulse in the rest of the ingredients.
5. Drop the combination onto the baking sheet in a rounded spoonful.
6. Bake for 20 to 25 minutes or wait until browned, flipping once halfway through.

Nutrition:

Calories 100

Fat 4.5g

Protein 6g

Net Carbs 4g

Bacon-Wrapped Shrimp

Preparation Time: 10 Minutes

Cooking Time: 15 Minutes

Servings: 4

Ingredients:

- Six slices of uncooked bacon
- Salt and pepper
- 12 large shrimp, peeled and deveined
- Paprika to taste

Directions:

1. Preheat the oven to 425 F

2. Cut the bacon in half, then wrap one piece around each shrimp.

3. Place the shrimp on the baking sheet and sprinkle with paprika, salt, and pepper.

4. Spray lightly with cooking spray, then bake for 15 minutes until bacon is crisp.

Nutrition:

Calories 100

Fat 6g

Protein 9g

Net Carbs 0.5g

Raspberry Cheesecake Fluff

Preparation Time: 5 Minutes

Cooking Time: 0 Minutes

Servings: 4

Ingredients:

- 1 cup heavy (whipping) cream

- 8 ounces cream cheese, at room temperature

- 4 ounces raspberries

- ½ cup sugar substitute (such as Swerve)

- One teaspoon vanilla extract

- Pinch salt

Directions:

1. In a blender or a bowl using a hand mixer, whip the cream to stiff peaks, 2 to 4 minutes.

2. Add the cream cheese, raspberries, sugar

substitute, vanilla, salt, and blend until smooth and well combined.

Nutrition:

Calories: 417

Total Fat: 41g

Protein: 5g

Total Carbs: 7g

Cholesterol: 143mg

Keto Hot Fudge

Preparation Time: 5 Minutes

Cooking Time: 10 Minutes

Servings: 10

Ingredients:

- ½ cup (1 stick) salted butter
- 4 ounces dark chocolate (85% or higher)
- Two tablespoons unsweetened cocoa powder
- 1 cup sugar substitute (such as Swerve)
- 1 cup heavy (whipping) cream
- Two teaspoons vanilla extract
- Pinch salt

Directions:

1. In a saucepan, dissolve the butter and chocolate. Add the cocoa powder and sweetener, and whisk until the powder and sweetener dissolve 3 to 5 minutes.

2. Add the cream and bring to a boil, stirring constantly. Reduce the heat to low, and add the vanilla and salt.

3. Remove from the heat, let rest for 5 minutes, and serve hot over your favorite dessert.

Nutrition:

Calories: 237 Total Fat: 24g

Protein: 2g Total Carbs: 5g

Fiber: 2g Cholesterol: 57mg

Hot Caramel Sauce

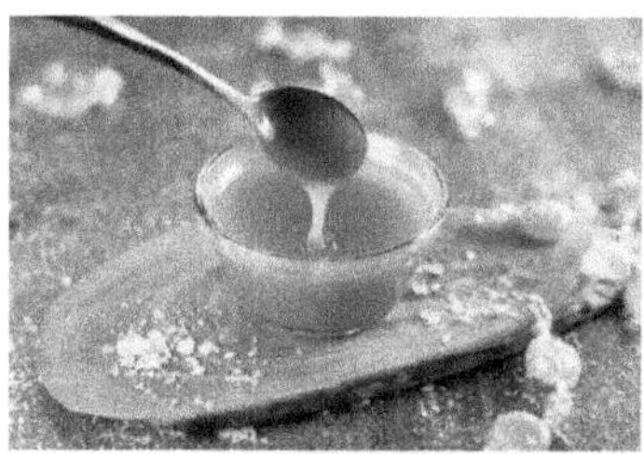

Preparation Time: 5 Minutes

Cooking Time: 10 Minutes

Servings: 8

Ingredients:

- ½ cup (1 stick) salted butter
- ¼ cup sugar substitute (such as Swerve)
- 1 cup heavy (whipping) cream
- ¼ to ½ teaspoon xanthan gum
- ½ teaspoon salt

Directions:

1. In a large saucepan over medium-low heat, dissolve the butter. Whisk in the sugar substitute until it is dissolved and incorporated, 3 to 5 minutes.
2. Add the cream, xanthan gum, and salt to the mixture, whisking continuously. Bring to a boil and let boil for 1 minute, then remove from the heat.
3. Serve hot.

Nutrition:

Calories: 202

Total Fat: 22g

Protein: 1g

Total Carbs: 1g

Cholesterol: 71mg

5-Minute Chocolate Mousse

Preparation Time: 5 Minutes

Cooking Time: 0 Minutes

Servings: 4

Ingredients:

- 1 (14-ounce) can coconut cream, chilled
- Three tablespoons unsweetened cocoa powder
- ¼ cup sugar substitute (such as Swerve)
- One teaspoon vanilla extract

Directions:

1. In a large mixing bowl, lash the coconut cream with a hand mixer until fluffy, about 3 minutes. If you don't have a hand mixer, you can whip it in the blender.
2. Fold in the cocoa powder, sugar substitute, and vanilla and serve immediately.

Nutrition:

Calories: 222

Total Fat: 22g

Protein: 1g

Total Carbs: 5g

Cholesterol: 0mg

Pumpkin Mousse

Preparation Time: 10 Minutes

Cooking Time: 30 Minutes

Servings: 4

Ingredients:

- 8 ounces cream cheese, at room temperature
- 1 cup canned pumpkin purée
- 1 cup heavy (whipping) cream
- Two tablespoons sugar substitute (such as Swerve)
- One teaspoon vanilla extract
- One teaspoon pumpkin pie spice
- ½ teaspoon ground cinnamon

Directions:

1. In a large mixer or a large bowl with a hand mixer, cream together the cream cheese and pumpkin until smooth, 1 to 2 minutes. If you don't have either type of mixer, you can use a blender.
2. Add the cream, sweetener, vanilla, pumpkin pie spice, and cinnamon. Mix it on high for 3 to 5 minutes, or until fluffy.
3. Chill for 30 minutes before serving.

Nutrition:

Calories: 419

Total Fat: 41g

Protein: 6g

Total Carbs: 9g

Cholesterol: 144mg

Snickerdoodle Mug Cake

Preparation Time: 5 Minutes

Cooking Time: 2 Minutes

Servings: 2

Ingredients:

- Two tablespoons salted butter
- Two tablespoons sugar substitute (such as Swerve)
- Two tablespoons almond flour
- Two tablespoons heavy (whipping) cream or coconut cream
- 1 large egg
- One teaspoon ground cinnamon, plus more for serving
- ½ teaspoon vanilla extract
- ½ teaspoon baking powder
- ¼ teaspoon cream of tartar
- ¼ teaspoon salt (optional)
- Cinnamon, for sprinkling

Directions:

1. In a coffee mug or glass measuring cup, microwave the butter until melted, about 30 seconds. Add the sugar substitute and stir vigorously with a fork. Add the almond flour, cream, egg, cinnamon, vanilla, baking powder, tartar, salt (if using), and mix until everything is combined.

2. Microwave for 50 to 70 seconds, or until the middle of the cake is

moist; careful not to overcook. Sprinkle with cinnamon and serve.

Nutrition:

Calories: 229 Total Fat: 23g

Protein: 5g Total Carbs: 2g

Cholesterol: 145mg

Chocolate Chip Cookie Skillet

Preparation Time: 10 Minutes

Cooking Time: 25 Minutes

Servings: 8

Ingredients:

- Olive oil cooking spray, for preparing the skillet
- 1 cup almond flour
- ½ cup coconut flour
- ½ teaspoon baking soda
- 1 teaspoon salt
- ½ cup coconut oil, at room temperature
- ¼ cup sugar substitute (such as Swerve)
- 1 large egg
- One teaspoon vanilla extract
- 1 cup sugar-free chocolate chips

Directions:

1. Preheat the oven to 350 F
2. Spray a 9-inch cast-iron skillet, pie dish, or cake pan with cooking spray or grease it with coconut oil.
3. In a large bowl, beat the almond flour, coconut flour, baking soda, and salt. Add the coconut oil, sugar substitute, egg, and vanilla, and whisk until combined. Fold in the chocolate

chips. Pour the batter into the prepared skillet.

4. Bake it for 20 to 25 minutes, or wait until brown on the edges and gooey in the center.

5. Let sit for 5 to 10 minutes. Serve warm.

Nutrition:

Calories: 390 Total Fat: 30g

Protein: 7g Total Carbs: 25g

Cholesterol: 33mg

Peanut Butter Fat Bombs

Preparation Time: 15 Minutes

Cooking Time: 1 Minute

Servings: 10

Ingredients:

- Two tablespoons coconut oil
- Two tablespoons salted butter
- ¼ cup peanut butter
- ¼ cup sugar substitute (such as Swerve)
- Two teaspoons vanilla extract
- Two tablespoons cream cheese

Directions:

1. In a medium, microwave-safe bowl, put the coconut oil, butter, peanut butter, sugar substitute, vanilla, and cream cheese. Microwave in 15-second increments, stirring in between until everything is melted and combined.

2. Pour the mixture into an ice cube tray or mini cupcake pan, and freeze for at least 4 hours.

3. Remove from the molds. Store it in an airtight vessel or a resealable plastic bag in the freezer for up to 3 months.

Nutrition:

Calories: 94

Total Fat: 9g

Protein: 2g

Total Carbs: 1g

Cholesterol: 9mg

CHAPTER 9:

Dinner

Grilled Leg of Lamb

Preparation Time: 5 Minutes

Cooking Time: 30 Minutes

Servings: 10

Ingredients:

- 1/3 cup olive oil
- ¼ cup fresh lemon juice
- Six garlic cloves, chopped
- ½ cup fresh oregano, chopped
- Salt and ground black pepper, as required
- One 4½-pounds grass-fed boneless leg of lamb, trimmed and butterflied

Directions:

1. In a shallow glass baking dish, mix well oil, lemon juice, garlic, oregano, salt, and black pepper.
2. Add the leg of lamb and generously coat with the mixture.
3. Cover the baking dish and refrigerate to marinate overnight, flipping occasionally.
4. Preheat the charcoal grill to medium-high heat. Grease the grill grate.
5. Remove the leg of the lamb from the refrigerator.

6. Carefully insert a long metal skewer crosswise in the butterflied leg.

7. Place leg of lamb onto the grill and cook for about 20-30 minutes, flipping occasionally.

8. Remove from the oven and place the leg of lamb over a cutting board.

9. With a piece of foil, cover the leg loosely for about 5-10 minutes before slicing.

10. With a sharp knife, cut the leg of lamb into desired size slices and serve.

Nutrition:

Calories: 452 Carbs: 1.5g

Carbohydrate: 3.1g

Fiber: 1.6g

Protein: 57.9g

Herb-Simmered Beef Stew

Preparation Time: 5 Minutes

Cooking Time: 55 Minutes

Servings: 6

Ingredients:

- Two teaspoons lard, at room temperature
- 1 ½ pounds top chuck, cut into bite-sized cubes
- 1 celery stalk, chopped
- 2 Italian peppers, chopped
- 1/2 cup onions, chopped
- Kosher salt, to season
- 1/4 teaspoon freshly cracked black pepper
- Two ripe tomatoes, pureed
- 4 cups vegetable broth
- 1 sprig thyme
- 1 sprig rosemary

- 1 bay laurel
- Two tablespoons fresh chives, roughly chopped

Directions:

1. Melt the lard in a soup pot over medium-high heat. Sear the top chuck cubes for 8 to 9 minutes until brown; reserve, keeping it warm.

2. Then, in the pan drippings, sauté the celery, Italian peppers, and onions for 5 minutes until they have softened. Add in the garlic, then continue to sauté for 30 seconds to 1 minute longer or until aromatic.

3. Add the kept beef back to the pot along with the salt, black pepper, tomatoes, vegetable broth, thyme, rosemary, and bay laurel.

4. Bring to a boil and immediately turn the heat to medium-low. Allow it to cook, partially covered, for 35 minutes longer.

5. Garnish with fresh chives and serve in individual bowls. Bon appétit!

Nutrition:

Calories 277

Fat 21.5g

Carbs 2.7g

Protein; 17.4g

Fiber 0.8g

Sesame and Chorizo Cauliflower Rice

Preparation Time: 5 Minutes

Cooking Time: 12 Minutes

Servings: 2

Ingredients:

- 8 oz grated cauliflower
- 2 oz chorizo
- 1/3 tsp ginger powder
- 1/3 tsp garlic powder
- 1 tbsp sesame oil

Seasoning:

- 1/3 tsp salt
- ¼ tsp ground black pepper
- 1 tbsp avocado oil

Directions:

1. Take a medium skillet pan, place it over medium heat, add avocado oil and when hot, add chorizo and cook for 3 to 5 minutes until thoroughly cooked.

2. Transfer chorizo to a plate, wipe clean the pan, return it over medium heat, add sesame oil and when hot, add grated cauliflower and cook 3 minutes until almost cooked.

3. Return chorizo into the pan, season with salt and black pepper, toss until mixed and then continue cooking for 2 to 3 minutes until thoroughly cooked.

4. Distribute chorizo cauliflower rice between two plates, top with sesame seeds, and then serve.

Nutrition:

Calories 229

Fats 20.5g

Protein 6.2g

Net Carb 1.4g

Fiber 2g

Cheddar Zucchini & Beef Mugs

Preparation Time: 5 Minutes

Cooking Time: 10 Minutes

Servings: 2

Ingredients:

- 4 oz roast beef deli slices, torn apart
- 3 tbsp sour cream
- One small zucchini, chopped
- 2 tbsp chopped green chilies
- 3 oz shredded cheddar cheese

Directions:

1. Divide the beef slices at the bottom of 2 wide mugs and spread tbsp of sour cream.
2. Top with two zucchini slices, season with salt and pepper, add green chilies, top with the remaining sour cream, and then cheddar cheese.
3. Place the mugs in the microwave for 1-2 minutes until the cheese melts.
4. Remove the mugs, let cool for 1 minute, and serve.

Nutrition:

Cal 188 Net Carbs 3.7g

Fat 9g Protein 18g

Grilled Beef Short Loin

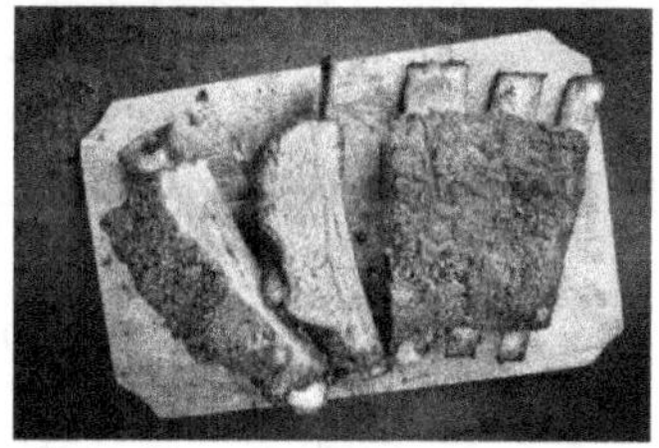

Preparation Time: 5 Minutes

Cooking Time: 30 Minutes

Servings: 3

Ingredients:

- 1 ½ pound beef short loin
- Two thyme sprigs, chopped
- One rosemary sprig, chopped
- 1 teaspoon garlic powder
- Sea salt and ground black pepper

Directions:

1. Place all of the above fixings in a re-sealable zipper bag. Shake until the short beef loin is well coated on all sides.
2. Cook on a preheated grill for 15 to minutes, flipping once or twice during the cooking time.
3. Let it sit for 5 minutes before slicing and serving. Bon appétit!

Nutrition: Calories 313

Fat 11.6g Carbs 0.1g

Protein 52g Fiber 0.1g

Herby Beef & Veggie Stew

Preparation Time: 5 Minutes

Cooking Time: 30 Minutes

Servings: 4

Ingredients:

- 1-pound ground beef

- 2 tbsp olive oil
- 1 onion, chopped
- Two garlic cloves, minced
- 14 ounces canned diced tomatoes
- 1 tbsp dried rosemary
- 1 tbsp dried sage
- 1 tbsp dried oregano
- 1 tbsp dried basil
- 1 tbsp dried marjoram
- Salt and black pepper, to taste
- Two carrots, sliced
- Two celery stalks, chopped
- 1 cup vegetable broth

Directions:

1. Set a pan over medium heat, add olive oil, onion, celery, garlic, and sauté for 5 minutes.

2. Place in the beef, and cook for 6 minutes.

3. Stir in the tomatoes, carrots, broth, black pepper, oregano, marjoram, basil, rosemary, salt, and sage, and simmer for minutes. Serve and enjoy!

Nutrition:

Cal 253 Fat 13g

Net Carbs 5.2g Protein 30g

Sausage with Zucchini Noodles

Preparation Time: 5 Minutes

Cooking Time: 12 Minutes

Servings: 2

Ingredients:

- One large zucchini, spiralized into noodles

- 3 oz sausage
- ½ tsp garlic powder
- 4 oz marinara sauce
- 2 tsp grated parmesan cheese

Seasoning:

- 1/3 tsp salt
- 1/8 tsp dried basil
- ¼ tsp Italian seasoning
- 1 tbsp avocado oil

Directions:

1. Take a skillet pan, place it over medium heat and hot, add sausage, crumble it and cook for 5 minutes until nicely browned.
2. When done, transfer sausage to a bowl, drain the grease, add oil and when hot, add zucchini noodles, sprinkle with garlic, toss until mixed, and cook for 3 minutes zucchini begins to tender.
3. Add marinara sauce, return sausage into the pan, toss until mixed, add salt, basil, and Italian seasoning, stir until mixed and cook for 2 to 3 minutes until hot.
4. When done, distribute marinara noodles between two plates, sprinkle with cheese, and then serve.

Nutrition:

Calories 320

Fats 27.6g

Protein 8.6g

Net Carb 5.2g

Fiber 2.7g

Ultimate Zucchini Lasagna

Preparation Time: 5 Minutes

Cooking Time: 45 Minutes

Servings: 7

Ingredients:

- Two tablespoons olive oil
- Sea salt and ground black pepper
- 2 ½ pounds ground chuck
- 1 shallot, chopped
- One teaspoon cayenne pepper
- One tablespoon steak seasoning blend
- One large-sized zucchini, sliced
- Seven eggs
- 7 ounces cream cheese
- 1 cup Asiago cheese, shredded

Directions:

1. Heat the olive oil with a moderate flame; once hot, brown the ground chuck for 4 to 5 minutes.

2. Add in the shallot and continue to sauté for 3 minutes more or until tender and translucent. Season with salt, black pepper, cayenne pepper, and steak seasoning blend.

3. Pat dry the zucchini slices to get rid of the excess moisture.

4. Spoon 1/3 of the combination into the bottom of a lightly greased casserole dish. Top with the layer of zucchini slices. Repeat until there is no zucchini and beef mixture.

5. In a mixing bowl, whisk the eggs with the sour cream; spread the mixture on top. Top with the Asiago cheese.

6. Cover the casserole dish with aluminum foil. Bake in the preheated oven at 3 degrees F for 20 minutes.

7. Remove the aluminum foil and bake for a further 15 minutes until the top is golden. Bon appétit!

Nutrition:

Calories 467

Fat 3.3g

Carbs 42g

Protein 42g

Fiber 0.4g

Tarragon Beef Meatloaf

Preparation Time: 5 Minutes

Cooking Time: 70 Minutes

Servings: 4

Ingredients:

- 2 lb. ground beef
- 3 tbsp flaxseed meal
- Two large eggs
- 2 tbsp olive oil
- 1 lemon, zested
- ¼ cup chopped tarragon
- ¼ cup chopped oregano
- Four garlic cloves, minced

Directions:

1. Preheat the oven to 400 F

2. Grease a loaf pan with cooking spray.

3. In a bowl, combine beef, salt, pepper, and

flaxseed meal; set aside.

4. In another bowl, whisk the eggs with olive oil, lemon zest, tarragon, oregano, and garlic. Pour the mixture onto the beef mix and evenly combine.

5. Spoon the meat mixture into the pan and press to fit in.

6. Bake in the oven for an hour.

7. Remove the pan, tilt to drain the meat's liquid, and let cool for 5 minutes.

8. Slice, garnish with some lemon slices and serve with curried cauli rice.

Nutrition:

Cal 631 Net Carbs 2.8g

Fat 38g Protein 64g

Sausage with Tomatoes and Cheese

Preparation Time: 5 Minutes

Cooking Time: 30 Minutes

Servings: 4

Ingredients:

- 2 ounces coconut oil, melted

- 2 pounds Italian pork sausage, chopped

- 1 onion, sliced

- Four sun-dried tomatoes, thinly sliced

- Salt and black pepper to the taste

- ½ pound gouda cheese, grated

- Three yellow bell peppers, chopped

- Three orange bell peppers, chopped

- A pinch of red pepper flakes
- Handful parsley, thinly sliced

Directions:

1. Warm a pan with medium-high heat, add sausage slices, stir, cook for 3 minutes on each side, transfer to a plate, and leave aside for now.
2. Heat the pan again over medium heat, add onion, yellow and orange bell peppers, and tomatoes, and stir and cook for 5 minutes.
3. Add pepper flakes and pepper, stir well, cook for 1 minute and take off the heat.
4. Arrange sausage slices into a baking dish, add bell peppers mix on top, add parsley and gouda, and introduce in the oven at 350 degrees F and bake for 15 minutes.
5. Divide between plates and serve hot.
6. Enjoy!

Nutrition:

Calories 200 Fat 5

Fiber 3 Carbs 6 Protein 14

Sweet & Sour Pork Chops

Preparation Time: 5 Minutes

Cooking Time: 50 Minutes

Servings: 6

Ingredients:

- Six 8-ounces ¾-inch thick pork shoulder chops, trimmed
- Salt and ground black pepper, as required

- Two tablespoons olive oil
- 1¼ cups water
- ¾ cup organic apple cider vinegar
- Six garlic cloves, mashed
- Two tablespoons Erythritol
- Two tablespoons fresh parsley, minced

Directions:

1. Preheat the oven to 400 degrees F.
2. Season each chop evenly with salt and black pepper.
3. In a large Dutch oven, heat the oil over high heat and sear the chops in 2 batches for about 5 minutes, flipping once halfway through.
4. Remove the pan from heat and arrange the chops in a single layer.
5. In a bowl, add the remaining fixings except for the parsley and mix well.
6. Add the vinegar mixture evenly over chops.
7. Cover the pan and transfer it into the oven.
8. Bake for about 40 minutes.
9. Garnish with parsley and serve hot.

Nutrition:

Calories: 777

Net Carbs: 1.3g

Carbohydrate: 1.4g

Fiber: 0.1g

Protein: 51.2g

Fat: 61.1g

Tuscan Pork Tenderloin with Cauli Rice

Preparation Time: 5 Minutes

Cooking Time: 30 Minutes

Servings: 4

Ingredients:

- 1 cup loosely packed fresh baby spinach
- 2 tbsp olive oil
- 1 ½ lb. pork tenderloin, cubed
- Salt and black pepper to taste
- ½ tsp cumin powder
- 2 cups cauliflower rice
- ½ cup of water
- 1 cup grape tomatoes, halved
- 3/4 cup crumbled feta cheese

Directions:

1. In a skillet, heat olive oil, season the pork with salt, pepper, and cumin, and sear on both sides for 5 minutes until brown.
2. Stir in cauli rice and pour in water. Cook for 5 minutes or until cauliflower softens.
3. Mix in spinach to wilt, minute, and add the tomatoes.
4. Spoon the dish into bowls, sprinkle with feta cheese, and serve with hot sauce.

Nutrition:

Cal 377

Net Carbs 1.9g

Fat 17g

Protein 43g

Baked Tenderloin with Lime Chimichurri

Preparation Time: 5 Minutes

Cooking Time: 1 Hour and 10 Minutes

Servings: 4

Ingredients:

- 1 lime, juiced
- ¼ cup chopped mint leaves
- ¼ cup rosemary, chopped
- Two cloves garlic, minced
- ¼ cup olive oil
- 4 lb. pork tenderloin
- Salt and black pepper to taste
- Olive oil for rubbing

Directions:

1. In a bowl, mix mint, rosemary, garlic, lime juice, olive oil, and salt, and combine well; set aside.

2. Preheat charcoal grill to 450 F, creating an immediate heat area and indirect heat area. Rub the pork using olive oil, season with salt and pepper.

3. Place the meat over direct heat and sear for 3 minutes on each side; then move to the indirect heat area.

4. Close the lid and cook for 25 minutes on one side, then open, flip, and the grill closed for 20 minutes.

5. Take away from the grill and let sit for 5 minutes before slicing. Spoon lemon chimichurri over the pork and serve.

Nutrition:

Cal 388

Net Carbs 2.1g

Fat 18g

Protein 28g

Shitake Butter Steak

Preparation Time: 5 Minutes

Cooking Time: 25 Minutes

Servings: 4

Ingredients:

- 2 cups shitake mushrooms, sliced
- Four ribeye steaks
- 2 tbsp butter
- 2 tsp olive oil
- Salt and black pepper to taste

Directions:

1. Heat olive oil in a pan with medium heat.
2. Rub the steaks with salt and pepper and cook for 4 minutes per side. Set aside.
3. Melt butter in the pan and cook the shitakes for 4 minutes.
4. Pour the butter and mushrooms over the steak.

Nutrition:

Cal 370 Net Carbs 3g

Fat 31g Protein 33g

Garlic and Lime Marinated Pork Chops

Preparation Time: 5 Minutes

Cooking Time: 10 Minutes

Servings: 2

Ingredients:

- Two pork chops
- 1 tsp minced garlic

- ¼ tsp cumin
- 1/3 tsp paprika
- ½ of lime, juiced, zested

Seasoning:

- ¼ tsp salt
- 1/8 tsp ground black pepper
- 1/3 tsp red chili powder

Directions:

1. Take a shallow dish, place all the ingredients in it except for pork and then stir until combined.
2. Add pork chops, toss until coated, and marinate for minutes in the refrigerator.
3. Then take a griddle pan, place it over medium-high heat, spray with oil, and when hot, place marinated pork chops

in it and grill for 4 to 5 minutes per side until thoroughly cooked.

4. Serve.

Nutrition:

Calories 180

Fats 8g

Protein 24.3 g

Net Carb 1.3g

Fiber 0.5g

Zoodles with Bolognese Sauce

Preparation Time: 5 Minutes

Cooking Time: 30 Minutes

Servings: 3

Ingredients:

- Three teaspoons olive oil
- 3/4-pound ground pork

- Two cloves garlic, pressed
- Two medium-sized tomatoes, pureed
- Two zucchinis, spiralized

Directions:

1. Heat oil in a saucepan with medium-high heat. Once hot, sear the pork for 3 to 4 minutes or until no longer pink.
2. Stir in the garlic and cook for 30 seconds more or until fragrant.
3. Fold in the pureed tomatoes and bring to a boil; immediately turn the heat to medium-low and continue simmering an additional 20 minutes.
4. After that, fold in the zoodles and continue to cook for a further 1 ½ minutes until just al dente. Serve hot. Bon appétit!

Nutrition:

Calories 357

Fat 28.7g

Carbs 4g

Protein 20.2g

Fiber 1.1g

Chili Zucchini Beef Lasagna

Preparation Time: 5 Minutes

Cooking Time: 55 Minutes

Servings: 4

Ingredients:

- ½ cup Pecorino Romano cheese
- Four yellow zucchinis, sliced

- Salt and black pepper to taste
- 1 tbsp lard
- ½ lb. ground beef
- 1 tsp garlic powder
- 1 tsp onion powder
- 2 tbsp coconut flour
- 1 ½ cups grated mozzarella
- 2 cups crumbled goat cheese
- 1 large egg
- 2 cups marinara sauce
- 1 tbsp Italian herb seasoning
- ¼ tsp red chili flakes
- ¼ cup fresh basil leaves

Directions:

1. Preheat oven to 375 F
2. Melt the lard in a skillet t and cook beef for minutes; set aside.
3. In a bowl, combine garlic powder, onion powder, coconut flour, salt, pepper, mozzarella cheese, half of Pecorino cheese, goat cheese, and egg.
4. Mix Italian herb seasoning and chili flakes with marinara sauce.
5. Make a single layer of the zucchini in a greased baking dish, spread ¼ of the egg mixture on top, and ¼ of the marinara sauce.
6. Repeat the process. Top it with the remaining Pecorino cheese.
7. Bake in the oven for 20 minutes. Garnish with basil, slice, and serve.

Nutrition:

Cal 608

Net Carbs 5.5g

Fat 37g

Protein 52g

Rib Roast with Roasted Red Shallots and Garlic

Preparation Time: 5 Minutes

Cooking Time: 55 Minutes

Servings: 6

Ingredients:

- 5 lb. beef rib roast, on the bone
- Three heads garlic, cut in half
- 3 tbsp olive oil
- Six shallots, peeled and halved
- Two lemons, zested and juiced

- 3 tbsp mustard seeds
- 3 tbsp swerve
- Salt and black pepper to taste
- 3 tbsp thyme leaves

Directions:

1. Preheat oven to 450°F. Place garlic heads and shallots in a roasting dish, toss with olive oil, and bake for minutes.

2. Pour lemon juice on them. Score shallow crisscrosses patterns on the meat and set aside.

3. Mix swerve, mustard seeds, thyme, salt, pepper, and lemon zest to make a rub; and apply it all over the beef.

4. Place the beef on the shallots and garlic; cook in the oven for 15 minutes. Reduce the heat to 400°F, cover the

dish with foil, and continue cooking for 5 minutes.

5. Once ready, remove the dish, and let sit covered for 15 minutes before slicing.

Nutrition:

Cal 556

Fat 38.6g

Net Carbs 2.5g

Protein 58.4g

Beef Ragù With A Twist

Preparation Time: 5 Minutes

Cooking Time: 25 Minutes

Servings: 6

Ingredients:

- 1 ½ pounds ground beef
- One bell pepper, deseeded and chopped
- 1 celery rib, chopped
- 1/2 cup shallots, chopped
- Two garlic cloves, chopped
- Two vine-ripe tomatoes, pureed
- 2 cups beef bone broth
- One tablespoon dried Italian herb seasoning

Directions:

1. In a lightly greased stockpot, brown the ground beef until no longer pink or about 5 minutes, crumbling with a spatula; reserve.

2. In the same pot, sauté the peppers, celery, and shallots, adding broth as needed. Continue to sauté until they have softened.

3. Now, stir in the garlic and continue to sauté for 40 seconds more. Add in the pureed tomatoes, beef bone broth, and Italian herb seasoning, bringing to a boil. Return the reserved beef to the pot.

4. Reduce heat to medium-low. Continue to simmer until the sauce has reduced to half of the volume or about 15 minutes. Bon appétit!

Nutrition:

Calories 349

Fat 21.8g

Carbs 4.9g

Protein 34g

Fiber 1.4g

Lemon Pork Chops with Buttered Brussels Sprouts

Preparation Time: 5 Minutes

Cooking Time: 27 Minutes

Servings: 6

Ingredients:

- 3 tbsp lemon juice
- Three cloves garlic, pureed
- 1 tbsp olive oil
- Six pork loin chops
- 1 tbsp butter
- 1 lb. brussels sprouts, trimmed and halved
- 2 tbsp white wine
- Salt and black pepper to taste

Directions:

1. Preheat broiler to 400°F and mix the lemon juice, garlic, salt, black

pepper, and oil in a bowl.

2. Brush the pork with the mixture, place on a baking sheet, and cook for 6 minutes on each side until browned.

3. Share into six plates and make the side dish.

4. Melt butter in a small wok or pan and cook in brussels sprouts for 5 minutes until tender.

5. Drizzle with white wine, sprinkle with salt and black pepper, and cook for another 5 minutes.

6. Ladle brussels sprouts to the side of the chops and serve with a hot sauce.

Nutrition:

Cal 549 Fat 48g

Net Carbs 2g

Protein 26g

Ground Pork & Scrambled Eggs with Cabbage

Preparation Time: 5 Minutes

Cooking Time: 30 Minutes

Servings: 4

Ingredients:

- 2 tbsp sesame oil
- Two large eggs
- 2 tbsp minced garlic
- ½ tsp ginger puree
- One medium white onion, diced
- 1 lb. ground pork
- One habanero pepper, chopped
- One green cabbage, shredded
- Five scallions, chopped
- 3 tbsp coconut aminos
- 1 tbsp white vinegar
- 2 tbsp sesame seeds

Directions:

1. Heat tbsp of sesame oil in a skillet over and scramble the eggs until set, 1 minute; set aside.
2. Heat 1 tbsp sesame oil in the same skillet and sauté garlic, ginger, and onion until soft and fragrant, 4 minutes.
3. Add ground pork and habanero pepper and season with salt, pepper. Cook for 10 minutes.
4. Mix in cabbage, scallions, aminos, and vinegar and cook until the cabbage is tender. Stir in the eggs.
5. Serve garnished with sesame seeds and some low carb tortillas.

Nutrition:

Cal 295

Net Carbs 3.6g

Fat 16g

Protein 29g

Cheeseburger Skillet with Bacon & Mushrooms

Preparation Time: 5 Minutes

Cooking Time: 20 Minutes

Servings: 4

Ingredients:

- Two slices Canadian bacon, chopped
- 1/2 cup shallots, sliced
- 1 garlic clove, minced
- 1-pound ground pork
- Sea salt and ground black pepper
- 1/3 cup vegetable broth

- 1/4 cup white wine
- 6 ounces Cremini mushrooms, sliced
- 1/2 cup cream cheese

Directions:

1. Heat a cast-iron skillet.
2. Cook the bacon and reserve the bacon and tablespoon of fat. Then, sauté the shallots and garlic in 1 tablespoon of bacon fat until tender and fragrant.
3. Add the ground pork, salt, and black pepper to the skillet. Cook for 4 to 5 minutes or until ground meat is nicely browned.
4. Add broth, wine, and mushrooms. Close the lid, then cook for 8 to 9 minutes over medium flame.
5. Turn off the heat. Add cream cheese and stir to combine. Serve topped with the reserved bacon. Enjoy!

Nutrition:

Calories 463

Fat 60g

Carbs 4.7g

Fiber 0.8g

Protein 36.2g

Traditional Beef Bourguignon

Preparation Time: 5 Minutes

Cooking Time: 1 Hour and 20 Minutes

Servings: 5

Ingredients:

- 1 ½ pounds shoulder steak, cut into cubes

- One tablespoon Herbs de Provence
- 1 onion, chopped
- 1 celery stalk, chopped
- 1 cup red Burgundy wine

Directions:

1. Heat a lightly greased soup pot over a medium-high flame. Now brown the beef in batches until no longer pink.
2. Add a splash of wine to deglaze your pan.
3. Add the Herbs de Provence, onion, celery, and wine to the pot; pour in cups of water and stir to combine well. Bring to a rapid boil; then, turn the heat to medium-low.
4. Close the lid and simmer for 1 hour 10 minutes. Serve over hot cauliflower rice if desired. Enjoy!

Nutrition:

Calories 217

Fat 5.5g

Carbs 3.9g

Protein 30g

Fiber 0.4g

Basil Prosciutto Pizza

Preparation Time: 5 Minutes

Cooking Time: 45 Minutes

Servings: 4

Ingredients:

- Four prosciutto slices, cut into thirds
- 2 cups grated mozzarella cheese
- 2 tbsp cream cheese, softened

- ½ cup almond flour
- 1 egg, beaten
- 1/3 cup tomato sauce
- 1/3 cup sliced mozzarella
- Six fresh basil leaves, to serve

Directions:

1. Preheat oven to 390 F
2. Microwave mozzarella cheese and 2 tbsp of cream cheese for a minute.
3. Mix in almond meal and egg.
4. Spread the mixture on the pizza pan and bake for 15 minutes; set aside.
5. Spread the tomato sauce on the crust. Arrange the mozzarella slices on the sauce and then the prosciutto.
6. Bake again for 15 minutes or wait until the cheese melts.
7. Remove and top with the basil. Slice and serve.

Nutrition:

Cal 160 Net Carbs 0.5g

Fats 6.2g

Protein 22g

Keto Crispy Rosemary Chicken Drumsticks

Preparation Time: 10 Minutes

Cooking Time: 40 Minutes

Servings: 4

Ingredients:

- 12 chicken drumsticks
- 4 tbsp. olive oil
- 4 tbsp. rosemary leaves
- 2 tsp. salt

Directions:

1. Preheat oven to 450 F.
2. Rub salt and rosemary on each chicken drumstick the blend and spot on a lubed heating plate.
3. Make sure the drumsticks are not contacting each other on the plate. Drizzle the olive oil or avocado oil over the chicken drumsticks.
4. Prepare for 40 minutes until the skin is firm.

Nutrition:

Calories 473

Fat 32 g

Carbs 6 g

Protein 42 g

Baked Pesto Chicken

Preparation Time: 5 Minutes

Cooking Time: 35 Minutes

Servings: 4

Ingredients:

- Four chicken breasts (about 1½ lb.)
- 3 tbsp. basil pesto
- 8 oz. mozzarella
- ½ tsp. salt
- ¼ tsp. black pepper

Directions:

1. Preheat oven to 350 F.
2. Coat heating dish with cooking spray. Put the chicken in the base in a single layer and sprinkle with the salt and pepper.
3. Spread the pesto on the bird. Put the mozzarella on top.
4. Heat for 35-45 minutes until the cheddar is bubbly.

5. Serve.

Nutrition:

Calories 471

Fat 22 g

Carbs 3.4 g

Protein 61 g

Low-Carb Pork Medallions

Preparation Time: 15 Minutes

Cooking Time: 20 Minutes

Servings: 2

Ingredients:

- 1 lb. pork tenderloin
- Three medium shallots
- ¼ cup oil

Directions:

1. Cut the meat into half-inch-thick slices.

2. Cleave the shallots and put them on a plate.

3. Warm the oil in a skillet.

4. Press each piece of pork into the shallots on both sides. The shallots will stick to the pork if you press firmly.

5. Put the meat slices, coated with shallots, into the warm oil and cook till carried out.

6. Some of the shallots will burn during cooking, but they'll give a heavenly taste to the red meat.

7. Simply cook the beef until it's cooked through.

8. Serve with vegetables.

Nutrition:

Calories 519 Fat 4 g

Carbs 7 g Protein 46 g

Keto Rosemary Roast Beef and White Radishes

Preparation Time: 10 Minutes

Cooking Time: 60 Minutes

Servings: 8

Ingredients:

- 3 lb. boneless beef roast
- Two white daikon radishes
- 3 tbsp. rosemary
- 2 tbsp. salt to taste
- 2 tbsp. olive oil

Directions:

1. Preheat oven to 400 F.
2. Spread olive oil, rosemary, and salt over the beef.
3. Put the stripped and severed radishes at the base of a warming dish.
4. Put the beef on the radishes and bake for one hour.
5. When done, wrap the burger in foil and let rest for 20 minutes before serving.

Nutrition:

Calories 492

Fat 39 g

Carbs 4.1 g

Protein 29 g

Bacon-Wrapped Pork Chops

Preparation Time: 10 Minutes

Cooking Time: 30 Minutes

Servings: 4

Ingredients:

- 12 oz. bacon package

- 6 to 8 boneless pork chops
- Salt and pepper

Directions:

1. Preheat your oven to 350 F
2. On a plate or cutting board, layout the pork chops.
3. Wrap each piece of pork in uncooked bacon cuts.
4. Place each bacon-wrapped pork chop onto the baking sheet.
5. Crush extra pepper over the highest point of the now bacon-wrapped pork.
6. Heat them for 30 minutes, flipping them at the 15-minute imprint. Serve promptly and appreciate it!

Nutrition:

Calories 350

Fat 2.8 g

Carbs 2.4 g

Protein 8 g

Rosemary Chicken with Avocado Sauce

Preparation Time: 4 Minutes

Cooking Time: 18 Minutes

Servings: 4

Ingredients:

- 1 avocado, pitted
- ½ cup mayonnaise
- 3 tbsp. ghee
- Four chicken breasts
- Salt and black pepper to taste
- 1 cup rosemary, chopped
- ½ cup chicken broth

Directions:

1. Spoon avocado, mayonnaise, and salt into a food processor and puree until it is a smooth sauce. Season to taste with salt. Pour sauce into a jar and refrigerate.
2. Melt ghee in a large skillet, season chicken with salt and black pepper, and fry for 4 minutes on each side to a golden brown. Remove chicken to a plate.
3. Pour broth into the same skillet and add cilantro. Bring to simmer for 3 minutes and add chicken.
4. Cover and cook on low heat for 5 minutes until the liquid has reduced. Dish chicken only into serving plates and spoon the mayo-avocado sauce over. Serve warm with buttered green beans and baby carrots.

Nutrition:

Calories 398

Fat 32 g

Carbs 4 g

Protein 24g

Crispy Chicken Nuggets

Preparation Time: 5 Minutes

Cooking Time: 20 Minutes

Servings: 4

Ingredients:

- 2 tbsp. ranch dressing
- ½ cup almond flour
- 1 egg
- 2 tbsp. garlic powder

- Four chicken breasts, cubed
- Salt and black pepper to taste
- 1 tbsp. butter, melted

Directions:

1. Preheat oven to 400 F, then grease a baking dish with the butter.
2. In a bowl, combine salt, garlic powder, flour, and pepper, and stir. In a separate bowl, beat egg.
3. Add the chicken to the egg mixture, then coat with the flour mixture. Bake for 18-20 minutes, turning halfway through. Remove to paper towels, drain the excess grease, and serve with ranch dressing.

Nutrition:

Calories 473

Fat 31 g

Carbs 7.6 g

Protein 43 g

Zucchini & Bell Pepper Chicken Gratin

Preparation Time: 5 Minutes

Cooking Time: 40 Minutes

Servings: 5

Ingredients:

- One red bell pepper, sliced
- 1 zucchini, chopped
- Salt and black pepper to taste
- 1 tsp. garlic powder
- 1 tbsp. olive oil
- Five chicken breasts, skinless and boneless, sliced
- 1 tomato, chopped
- ½ tsp. dried oregano
- ½ tsp. dried basil

- ½ cup mozzarella cheese, shredded

Directions:

1. Coat the chicken with salt, black pepper, and garlic powder. Warm olive oil in a skillet over medium heat and add the chicken slices. Cook until golden and remove to a baking dish.

2. To the same pan, add the zucchini, tomato, bell pepper, basil, oregano, and salt, cook for 2 minutes, and spread over the chicken. Bake in the oven at 360 F for 20 minutes.

3. Sprinkle the mozzarella over the chicken, return to the oven, and bake for 5 minutes more until the cheese is melted and bubbling.

Nutrition:

Calories 467

Fat 23.5 g

Carbs 6.2 g

Protein 45.7 g

Coconut Chicken with Creamy Asparagus Sauce

Preparation Time: 5 Minutes

Cooking Time: 25 Minutes

Servings: 4

Ingredients:

- 2 tbsp. butter
- 1-pound chicken thighs
- 2 tbsp. coconut oil
- 2 tbsp. coconut flour
- 2 cups asparagus, chopped

- 1 tsp. oregano
- 1 cup heavy cream
- 1 cup chicken broth

Directions:

1. Heat a frypan over medium heat
2. Add the coconut oil to melt. Brown the chicken on all sides, approximately 6-8 minutes. Set aside.
3. Melt the butter and whisk in the flour over medium heat. Whisk in the heavy cream and chicken broth and bring to a boil. Stir in oregano.
4. Add the asparagus to the skillet, then cook for 10 minutes until tender. Handover to a food processor and pulse until smooth. Season with salt and pepper.

Return to the skillet and add the chicken; cook for 5 minutes and serve.

Nutrition.

Calories 451

Fat 36.7 g

Carbs 3.2 g

Protein 18.5 g

Herb Pork Chops with Cranberry Sauce

Preparation Time: 5 Minutes

Cooking Time: 2 Hours and 40 Minutes

Servings: 2

Ingredients:

- Four pork chops
- ½ tsp. garlic powder
- Salt and black pepper to taste

- 1 tsp. fresh basil, chopped
- A drizzle of olive oil
- ½ onion, chopped
- ½ cup white wine
- Juice of ½ lemon
- 1 bay leaf
- 1 cup chicken stock
- Fresh parsley, chopped, for serving
- 1 cup cranberries
- ½ tsp. fresh rosemary, chopped
- ½ cup xylitol
- ½ cup of water
- ½ tsp. harissa paste sriracha sauce

Directions:

1. Preheat oven to 360 F.
2. In a bowl, combine the pork chops with basil, salt, garlic powder, and black pepper. Heat a pan with a drizzle of oil over medium heat, put the pork in, and cook until browned, about 4-5 minutes; set aside.
3. Stir in the onion and cook for 2 minutes.
4. Next, you need to add the bay leaf and wine and cook for 4 minutes.
5. Pour in lemon juice and chicken stock and simmer for 5 minutes.
6. Return the pork and cook for 10 minutes. Cover the pan and put it in the oven for 2 hours.
7. Set a pan over medium-high heat, add the cranberries, rosemary, sriracha sauce, water, and xylitol, and bring to a simmer for 15 minutes.
8. Take away the pork chops from the oven and discard the bay leaf.

Pour the sauce over the pork and serve sprinkled with parsley.

Nutrition:

Calories 450

Fat 23.5 g

Carbs 7.3 g

Protein 42 g

Pork Chops with Basil Tomato Sauce

Preparation Time: 10 Minutes

Cooking Time: 40 Minutes

Servings: 4

Ingredients:

- Four pork chops
- ½ tbsp. fresh basil, chopped
- 1 garlic clove, minced
- 1 tbsp. olive oil
- 7 oz. canned diced tomatoes
- ½ tbsp. tomato paste
- Salt and black pepper to taste
- ½ red chili, finely chopped

Directions:

1. Season the pork with black pepper and salt. Set a pan over medium heat and warm oil, put in the pork chops, cook for 3 minutes, turn and cook for another 3 minutes; remove to a bowl. Add the garlic and cook for 30 seconds.

2. Stir in the tomato paste, tomatoes, and chili; bring to a boil, and reduce heat to medium-low. Put in the pork chops, cover the pan,

and simmer everything for 30 minutes. Remove the pork chops to plates and sprinkle with fresh oregano to serve.

Nutrition:

Calories 425

Fat 25 g

Carbs 2.5 g

Protein 39 g

Citrus Pork with Sautéed Cabbage & Tomatoes

Preparation Time: 7 Minutes

Cooking Time: 20 Minutes

Servings: 4

Ingredients:

- 3 tbsp. olive oil
- 2 tbsp. lemon juice
- 1 garlic clove, pureed
- Four pork loin chops
- 1/3 head cabbage, shredded
- 1 tomato, chopped
- 1 tbsp. white wine
- Salt and black pepper to taste
- ¼ tsp. cumin
- ¼ tsp. ground nutmeg
- 1 tbsp. parsley

Directions:

1. In a bowl, blend the lemon juice, garlic, salt, pepper, and olive oil. Brush the pork with the mixture.

2. Preheat grill to high heat. Grill the pork for 2-3 minutes on each side until cooked through. Remove to serving plates. Warm the remaining olive oil in a pan and cook cabbage for 5 minutes.

3. Drizzle with white wine, sprinkle with cumin, nutmeg, salt, and pepper. Add the tomatoes, then cook for another 5 minutes, stirring occasionally.

4. Spoon the sautéed cabbage to the side of the chops and serve sprinkled with parsley.

Nutrition:

Calories 565 Fat 36.7 g

Carbs 6.1 g Protein 43 g

Rosemary Buttered Pork Chops

Preparation Time: 5 Minutes

Cooking Time: 20 Minutes

Servings: 4

Ingredients:

- ½ tbsp. olive oil
- 2 tbsp. butter
- 1 tbsp. rosemary
- Four pork chops
- Salt and black pepper to taste
- Pinch of paprika
- ½ tsp. chili powder

Directions:

1. Rub the pork chops with olive oil, salt, black pepper, paprika, and chili powder. Heat a grill to medium, add the pork chops and cook for 10 minutes, flipping once halfway through.

2. Remove to a serving plate. In a pan over low heat, warm the butter until it turns a nutty brown. Pour over the pork chops, sprinkle with rosemary, and serve.

Nutrition:

Calories 363 Fat 21.4 g

Carbs 3.8 g

Protein 38.5 g

Beef Tenderloin

Preparation Time: 15 Minutes

Cooking Time: 15 Minutes

Servings: 4

Ingredients:

- 6 tbsp. Butter, salted, softened & divided
- 2 Garlic cloves, minced finely
- 4 oz. Mushrooms, chopped finely
- 1 tbsp. Avocado Oil
- 1 1/2 lbs. Beef Tenderloin Steaks, sliced
- Salt & Pepper, as needed

Directions:

1. First, spoon in two tablespoons of butter to a heated saucepan over medium-high heat.
2. Once the butter has melted, stir in the mushrooms.
3. Cook them for 4 minutes or until they are golden brown.
4. Now, stir in the garlic, salt, and pepper to it and sauté for a minute.
5. Move the mushrooms to a plate and set it aside.
6. With a fork, coat the mushrooms with the left butter.
7. After that, keep the butter in waxed paper and roll it into a log by wrapping it up. Chill it until it needs to be used.

8. Keep the steaks at room temperature about 2 hours before it is being cooked.

9. Then, take a large saucepan over medium-high heat, and to this, pour the oil.

10. When the oil is heated, stir in the steaks and cook for 5 minutes per side. Tip: If it is thicker, more time is needed.

11. Take the pan from heat and set it aside for 3 minutes or until the meat's internal temperature reaches 140F to 150F.

12. Serve warm with the chilled butter on top.

Nutrition:

Calories: 406Kcal

Carbohydrates: 2.3g

Fat: 24.1g Proteins: 38.1g

Buttered Chicken with Brussels Sprouts

Preparation Time: 5 Minutes

Cooking Time: 30 Minutes

Servings: 4

Ingredients:

- 8 Chicken Breasts
- Three cloves of Garlic cloves,
- minced finely
- 1 lb. Brussels sprouts,
- whole or sliced into half
- ¾ cup Chicken Broth
- ½ tsp. Sea Salt
- 2 tsp. Butter, preferably grass-fed
- ¼ tsp. Black Pepper

Directions:

1. Start by placing the chicken pieces in a heated, large saucepan over medium-high heat.

2. Now, spoon in salt and pepper over it. Sear it for 3 to 4 minutes or until the chicken is cooked and is slightly browned at the bottom.

3. Turn them over and top it with salt and pepper. Cook for a few minutes.

4. Put the cooked chicken to a plate and add the brussels sprouts to the pan.

5. Next, pour the chicken stock into it and allow it to simmer for about 10 minutes.

6. Return the chicken pieces to the heat and cook for a few minutes or until the chicken is fully cooked.

7. Finally, stir in the butter and garlic to the pan. Sauté the garlic for 2 minutes or until aromatic.

8. Spoon the garlic butter over the top of the chicken and brussels sprouts. Coat well and stir.

9. Transfer to the serving bowl and serve it hot. Garnish it with black pepper.

Nutrition:

Calories: 446Kcal

Carbohydrates: 8g Fat: 15.1

Proteins: 63.7g

Pork Stir-Fry

Preparation Time: 5 Minutes

Cooking Time: 20 Minutes

Servings: 4

Ingredients:

- 10 oz. Broccoli florets

- 2 tbsp. Sesame Oil
- 1 Carrot, sliced thinly into sticks
- 2 tbsp. Tamari
- 1 lb. Pork Tenderloin, sliced
- 2 Garlic cloves, minced
- ½ tsp. Ginger, fresh & minced

Directions:

1. First, spoon in the one tablespoon of oil to a large saucepan and heat it over medium-high heat.
2. Once the oil becomes hot, stir in the pork and cook for 6 minutes or until browned.
3. Then, pour the rest of the oil into the pan over high heat.
4. After that, add garlic and stir for 30 seconds or until fragrant.
5. Now, stir in the broccoli to it and mix well.
6. Continue cooking for 5 minutes or until tender and softened. Cover for further 2
7. minutes while keeping it covered.
8. Finally, return the pork to the pan and spoon in ginger and tamari sauce. Stir until the vegetables are prepared to your desire continuously.

Nutrition:

Calories: 247Kcal

Carbohydrates: 8g

Fat: 12g

Fiber: 3g

Saturated Fat: 2g

Sugar: 3g

Proteins: 27g

Sodium: 326m

Cauliflower Chowder

Preparation Time: 5 Minutes

Cooking Time: 25 Minutes

Servings: 4

Ingredients:

- 1 tbsp. Butter, preferably grass-fed
- 1 Cauliflower head, torn into florets
- ½ cup Onion, finely diced
- 1 ½ cups Vegetable Stock
- Five cloves of Garlic, finely minced
- ½ cup Carrots, diced
- Salt, to taste
- ¼ cup Cream cheese
- 1 tsp. Pepper, grounded freshly
- ½ tsp. Oregano, dried
- Olive Oil, as required

Directions:

1. Start by heating a Dutch oven medium heat, and stir in butter, onions, and garlic.
2. Cook for 4 minutes or wait until the onions are softened.
3. Next, stir in carrots, pepper, cauliflower, oregano, vegetable broth, and salt to the Dutch oven.
4. Bring the mixture to a boil and allow it to simmer. Reduce heat.
5. Simmer for 15 minutes or until the cauliflower is soft & cooked.
6. Remove from heat. With an immersion blender, blend the soup partly.
7. Now, return the soup to the stove. Pour a cup of

broth along with the cream cheese.

8. Combine.

9. Simmer for further 10 minutes. Drizzle with olive oil and serve it hot.

Nutrition:

Calories: 130Kcal

Carbohydrates: 10g

Fat: 7g

Proteins: 5g

Chicken Cobb Salad

Preparation Time: 10 Minutes

Cooking Time: 10 Minutes

Servings: 4

Ingredients:

- 1/2 lb. Chicken, sliced
- ¼ tsp. Smoked Paprika
- 2 Eggs, hardboiled & chopped
- 2 tbsp. Olive Oil
- Salt & Pepper, as needed
- 4 Ham slices
- ¼ tsp. Onion Powder
- ½ of 1 Avocado, medium & sliced
- ½ cup Cucumbers, chopped
- 3 cups Greens of your choice
- ½ cup Cherry Tomatoes quartered

Directions:

1. First, marinate the chicken with salt, onion powder, pepper, and smoked paprika. Set it aside.

2. Heat a large cast-iron skillet over medium-low heat.

3. Stir in the chicken and sear it for 4 minutes on each side or until the

chicken is cooked. Slice it once cooled.

4. Place all the remaining ingredients needed to make the salad along with the chicken.

5. Serve it with the dressing just before serving.

6. Enjoy.

Nutrition:

Calories: 130Kcal

Proteins: 5g

Fiber: 4g

Fat: 7g Carbohydrates:

Sugar: 4g

Sodium: 454mg

Cauliflower Pizza

Preparation Time: 10 Minutes

Cooking Time: 30 Minutes

Servings: 6

Ingredients:

- 1 Cauliflower head, mcdium & finely chopped
- 1 cup Mozzarella Cheese, grated
- 1 Egg, large & preferably farm-raised
- Salt & Pepper, to taste

Directions:

1. First, place the cauliflower chops in the food processor and process them until they are riced. Tip: Do not over process and puree it.

2. Next, transfer the riced cauliflower to a glass bowl and microwave them for 5 minutes or until they are soft.

3. After that, move the softened cauliflower to a clean tea towel and

squeeze it well to remove all the moisture. Tip: It should not have any moisture as the pizza crust won't be crispy then.

4. Now, keep the squeezed cauliflower in a large-sized bowl and stir in the egg, grated cheese, and seasoning to it.

5. Combine well until you get a cauliflower dough.

6. Then, transfer the cauliflower 'dough' to a parchment-paper-lined baking sheet and spread it out evenly.

7. Apply olive oil over the cauliflower crust and bake at 180 C or 350 F for 14 minutes or until golden in color.

8. Finally, top it with toppings of your choice and garnish with more cheese.

9. Bake for further 5 minutes or until the cheese is gooey and bubbling.

10. Serve it hot.

Nutrition:

Calories: 236Kcal

Carbohydrates: 4g Fat: 15.5g

Proteins: 17.8g

Sirloin Steak

Preparation Time: 10 Minutes

Cooking Time: 13 Minutes

Servings: 4

Ingredients:

- 4 × 8 oz. Sirloin Steak
- 1 tbsp. Butter, preferably
- grass-fed
- For the marinade:

- ¼ cup Coconut Aminos
- ½ tsp. Black Pepper
- ¼ cup Olive Oil
- 1 tsp. Sea Salt
- 2 tbsp. Balsamic Vinegar
- ½ tsp. Garlic Powder
- 1 tsp. Italian Seasoning

Directions:

1. First, marinate the steak with the marinade and allow it to marinate overnight if time permits.
2. Before cooking, thaw the meat about half an hour before.
3. Preheat the oven to 200 C or 400 F.
4. Meanwhile, heat a large cast-iron skillet over medium-high heat.
5. Now, spoon in the butter and melt it.
6. Then, place the steaks in a single layer in the skillet and sear them for 2 to 3 minutes per side or until they are browned with grill marks.
7. Next, transfer the skillet to the oven. Bake for 3 to 6 minutes or until it is cooked to your desired doneness.
8. Take the skillet from the oven. Allow it to cool for 5 minutes before slicing.
9. Serve it warm.

Nutrition:

Calories: 475Kcal

Carbohydrates: 5g Fat: 26g

Fiber: 0g Saturated Fat: 9g

Sugar: 1g Proteins: 49g

Sodium: 554mg

Bacon-Wrapped Chicken

Preparation Time: 5 Minutes

Cooking Time: 20 Minutes

Servings: 4

Ingredients:

- 1 lb. Chicken Breast Tenderloin
- 8 Bacon Slices
- 4 Aged Cheddar Cheese Slices, sliced into two

Directions:

1. First, to make this easy chicken fare, pour water into a large mixing bowl filled with warm water and spoon in salt. Mix.
2. Next, place the chicken breast tenderloin in it and soak it for a minimum of 10 minutes.
3. Tip: The chicken should be immersed in it.
4. Preheat the oven to 230 C
5. Now, take out the chicken from the water and dry it up using a paper towel.
6. Then, make a slice in the middle of the chicken pieces and place the cheese slices.
7. After that, wrap the bacon over the stuffed chicken.
8. Once covered, arrange the chicken pieces on a greased parchment-paper-lined baking sheet.
9. Finally, bake for about 15minutes or until the chicken is cooked through.

10. When done, keep the chicken pieces under the broiler for 2 to 3 minutes to become crispier.

Nutrition:

Calories: 301Kcal

Carbohydrates: 1g

Fat: 17g

Proteins: 35g

Pork Tenderloin

Preparation Time: 10 Minutes

Cooking Time: 20 Minutes

Servings: 8

Ingredients:

- 1 lb. × 2 Pork Tenderloins
- ½ tsp. Oregano, dried
- 1 tbsp. Olive Oil
- 1 tbsp. Dijon Mustard
- For the sauce:
- 1 tsp. Tarragon
- ¼ tsp. Garlic Powder
- 2 tsp. Hot Horseradish
- 1 cup Chicken Stock
- Salt & Pepper, as required
- 1/3 cup Heavy Cream
- 1 tbsp. Dijon Mustard
- 1 tbsp. Butter, preferably grass-fed

Directions:

1. To begin with, slice each of the pork tenderloins into three pieces.

2. With the help of a meat mallet, pound the meat pieces until ½ thick. Place it in a large wide plate.

3. Now, spoon in olive oil, pepper, oregano, and Dijon mustard. Set it aside for 15 minutes.

4. In the meantime, place all the ingredients needed to make the sauce, excluding butter, in a frying pan.

5. Bring the sauce to a boil, then lower the heat. Simmer the mixture for 12 minutes or until thickened.

6. Off the heat and spoon in the butter to it. Whisk well.

7. Preheat the grill to high heat.

8. Arrange the pork pieces on high heat and grill for 4 minutes per side or until it is slightly pink inside.

9. Keep it aside for 5 minutes.

10. Serve it warm and drizzle the sauce over it. Enjoy.

Nutrition:

Calories: 229Kcal

Carbohydrates: 0.01g

Fat: 11g

Proteins: 24g

Conclusion

Keto can be a great option for people looking to shed extra weight that is stored in their bodies as fat.

Ketosis is the process of the body using fats instead of glucose for energy. The liver can take fats and break them down into ketones, which can be used by both the body and the brain as a fuel source. To get the body away from using sugars, however, a person has to severely limit the amount and type of carbs they consume so the body can burn through its glucose stores and start working on the fat stores. This is why it can be so important to stay diligent on the diet once started; otherwise, a person might not see their desired results.

For people who are ready to dedicate themselves 100% to the keto diet, there are various forms of it that can match any person's lifestyle and goals. The standard keto option is best for people trying the diet for the first time because it can be the quickest way to get into ketosis and reap the immediate benefits. There are also cyclical and targeted keto for people who might not be willing to follow the strict diet every day. These options give people an opportunity to consume carbs on certain days based on their own personal plans.

There are many benefits to starting the keto diet beyond just losing weight. Keto can also help people improve their heart health by reducing bad fats and forcing the body to work through fats it has stored, possibly in dangerous places like arteries. It can also help people with certain types of epilepsy reduce seizures by switching the brain onto ketone power. Keto can also help women with PCOS regain their health by promoting weight loss and helping to balance their hormones, which can be a cause of the condition. It can even help clear up acne in some people by reducing blood sugar, which can improve skin conditions.

Keeping keto long term can seem difficult for beginners who are just getting used to the mechanics of the diet, but it is not so difficult once they are acclimated to the keto lifestyle. Planning out meals and snacks can help people keep up keto longer because it takes some of the work and thinking out of dieting. A person can simply grab what they need and go. And if the standard keto doesn't work for someone long term, they can refer to the other keto styles to find one that will work for them beyond the initial diet.

Lastly, I wish that you will be able to achieve your desired weight and at the same time enjoy the keto diet experience with these recipes. Happy eating!